g.uk/libr

D1766269

BRITISH MEDICAL ASSOCIATION

0778340

Practical Guide to Neurovascular Emergencies

Guillaume Saliou · Marie Théaudin
Claire Join-Lambert Vincent
Raphaëlle Souillard-Scemama

Practical Guide to
Neurovascular Emergencies

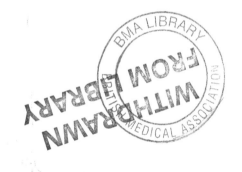

BMA LIBRARY
BRITISH MEDICAL ASSOCIATION
WITHDRAWN FROM LIBRARY

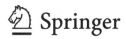

Springer

Guillaume Saliou
Service de neurologie
Hôpital du Kremlin-Bicêtre
Le Kremlin-Bicêtre
France

Raphaëlle Souillard-Scemama
Service de neuroradiologie
Centre hospitalier Sainte-Anne
Paris
France

Claire Join-Lambert Vincent
Service de neurologie
Hôpital Saint Joseph
Paris
France

Marie Théaudin
Service de neurologie
Hôpital du Kremlin-Bicêtre
Le Kremlin-Bicêtre
France

ISBN 978-2-8178-0480-4   ISBN 978-2-8178-0481-1   (eBook)
DOI 10.1007/978-2-8178-0481-1
Springer Paris Heidelberg New York Dordrecht London

Library of Congress Control Number: 2013940752

Translation from the French language edition 'Guide pratique des urgences neurovasculaires' by Guillaume Saliou, Marie Théaudin, Claire Join-Lambert Vincent, Raphaëlle Souillard-Scemama, © Springer-Verlag France, Paris, 2010; ISBN: 978-2-8178-0177-3.

© Springer-Verlag France 2014
This work is subject to copyright. All rights are reserved by the Publisher, whether the whole or part of the material is concerned, specifically the rights of translation, reprinting, reuse of illustrations, recitation, broadcasting, reproduction on microfilms or in any other physical way, and transmission or information storage and retrieval, electronic adaptation, computer software, or by similar or dissimilar methodology now known or hereafter developed. Exempted from this legal reservation are brief excerpts in connection with reviews or scholarly analysis or material supplied specifically for the purpose of being entered and executed on a computer system, for exclusive use by the purchaser of the work. Duplication of this publication or parts thereof is permitted only under the provisions of the Copyright Law of the Publisher's location, in its current version, and permission for use must always be obtained from Springer. Permissions for use may be obtained through RightsLink at the Copyright Clearance Center. Violations are liable to prosecution under the respective Copyright Law. The use of general descriptive names, registered names, trademarks, service marks, etc. in this publication does not imply, even in the absence of a specific statement, that such names are exempt from the relevant protective laws and regulations and therefore free for general use.
While the advice and information in this book are believed to be true and accurate at the date of publication, neither the authors nor the editors nor the publisher can accept any legal responsibility for any errors or omissions that may be made. The publisher makes no warranty, express or implied, with respect to the material contained herein.

Printed on acid-free paper

Springer is part of Springer Science+Business Media (www.springer.com)

Foreword

A group of four young neuroradiologists and neurologists (Guillaume Saliou, Marie Théaudin, Claire Join-Lambert and Raphaëlle Souillard-Scemama) has rightly placed neuroimaging at the very heart of this book on neurovascular emergencies, as no evidence-based emergency treatment is available for subjects with sudden onset of hemiplegia or aphasia without at least one preliminary CT scan to exclude cerebral haemorrhage. This is so true that trials of brain CT in the ambulance are currently underway, as *time is brain*: one patient out of four recovers without sequelae when thrombolysis is performed within the first 90 min following onset of symptoms, versus one out of fourteen patients treated between three and four and a half hours. The authors have rightly emphasized the role of MRI, as although brain CT is able to exclude cerebral haemorrhage, visualize cerebral arteries by means of CT angiography and even allows increasingly accurate assessment of cerebral perfusion, it does not provide the fundamental information available with diffusion-weighted MRI with calculation of the apparent diffusion coefficient to assess viability of brain tissue.

Apart from management in the stroke unit, which has been demonstrated for a long time to be effective in all types of stroke, progress in imaging and treatment has essentially concerned cerebral ischaemia and the authors have therefore devoted the major part of the book to this disease. However, they have not neglected clinical features that are briefly summarized underneath each image and in each chapter, or cerebral and meningeal haemorrhage and even long-term sequelae such as superficial haemosiderosis, and rare spinal cord vascular diseases. The authors also had the original idea to discuss a number of complex and relatively common situations, such as incidentalomas, white matter hyperintensity, aneurysms, venous developmental anomalies, etc. They also discuss various "stroke mimics", such as tumours, multiple sclerosis and infections.

This book does not claim to be comprehensive and the order of the chapters may appear somewhat surprising, as it could be argued that thrombolysis could have been discussed before the last chapter or that certain aspects of cerebro-vascular disease are discussed in more detail than others. This handbook will nevertheless be very useful to neuroradiologists and neurologists in their daily practice and more widely to all physicians who manage patients with cerebro-vascular disease.

The authors' enthusiasm, their original approach, the wealth and quality of imaging would certainly have pleased the late Pierre LASJAUNIAS who was the department head for two of the authors and who made a major contribution to the management of cerebrovascular disease in France and abroad and to the reputation of Bicêtre hospital. These four young authors have paid him a great tribute with this book.

Prof. Marie-Germaine Bousser

Contents

Abbreviations

ACA	Anterior cerebral artery
ADC	Apparent diffusion coefficient
AICA	Anterior inferior cerebellar artery
APS	Antiphospolipid syndrome
APTT	Activated partial thromboplastin time
AVM	Arteriovenous malformation
CBF	Cerebral blood flow
CBV	Cerebral blood volume
CRP	C-Reactive protein and IA Intra Arterial
CSF	Cerebrospinal fluid
DIC	Disseminated intravascular coagulation
ENT	Ear, nose and throat
FDP	Fibrinogen degradation product
GE	Gradient echo
LVEF	Left ventricular ejection fraction
MCA	Middle cerebral artery
MTT	Mean transit time
NIHSS	National Institutes of Health Stroke Scale
PCA	Posterior cerebral artery
PICA	Posterior inferior cerebellar artery
PT	Prothrombin Time
SAT	Supra-aortic trunks
SE	Spin echo
SLE	Systemic Lupus erythematosus
TIA	Transient ischaemic attack
TMA	Thrombotic microangiopathy
TOE	Transoesophageal echocardiography
TTE	Transthoracic echocardiography
VKA	Vitamin K antagonist

Introduction

This book is the fruit of a collaboration between neurologists and neuroradiologists.

Each of these specialties has its own vision of cerebrovascular disease and is used to working according to different approaches. We have endeavoured to meet the expectations of these two specialties so that clinicians as well as radiologists can easily find answers to their everyday questions in neurovascular disease.

This book does not claim to be exhaustive. With its pocket book format, it is designed to be an easily accessible tool for clinicians and radiologists involved in the management of patients with central nervous system vascular disease.

At the acute phase of stroke, after performing physical examination, radiological investigations play a decisive role in the treatment strategy. Based on imaging, we describe the management plans and treatment (in line with current guidelines) for each situation encountered in neurovascular disease.

Ischemic strokes can present a wide range of radiological signs depending on the arterial territory and the size of the vessels involved, in contrast with haemorrhagic strokes, associated with fewer radiological signs. Consequently, a large part of this book is devoted to cerebral infarction with a briefer discussion of cerebral haemorrhage.

The aim of this book, for the various specialists involved in the management of neurovascular disease, is therefore to integrate imaging at an earlier stage of the clinical assessment and to include clinical findings in the radiological assessment.

Chapter 1
Principles of Magnetic Resonance Imaging

Classical Neuroimaging Sequences

FLAIR (Fig. 1.1)

T2-weighted fluid-attenuated inversion-recovery (FLAIR) sequences suppress the free water signal, such as that of cerebrospinal fluid (CSF), giving a markedly hypointense signal. However, the signal of oedema containing bound water is not suppressed and gives a hyperintense signal.

MRI abnormalities are observed from about the 3rd hour after onset of arterial ischaemia.

T2-Weighted Gradient-Echo

Synonyms: T2-weighted gradient-echo, T2-GE, T2*, T2-star (Fig. 1.1).

T2- and T1-weighted gradient-echo sequences are very sensitive to magnetic susceptibility artifacts.

Methaemoglobin contains iron, which induces artifacts. These sequences are therefore widely used to detect a haemorrhagic component within a zone of infarction or old haemorrhage. Blood has a markedly hypointense signal. This sequence is also useful to demonstrate intravascular thrombus, particularly venous thrombus in the context of cerebral venous thrombosis.

T2 and T1-Weighted Spin-Echo

Synonym: T2 and T1-SE (Fig. 1.2)

In addition to demonstrating signs of ischaemia about 3 h after onset of symptoms, as hypointensity on T1 and hyperintensity on T2, these sequences may also visualize arterial thrombus, as blood is markedly hypointense *(flow void)*,

G. Saliou et al., *Practical Guide to Neurovascular Emergencies*,
DOI: 10.1007/978-2-8178-0481-1_1, © Springer-Verlag France 2014

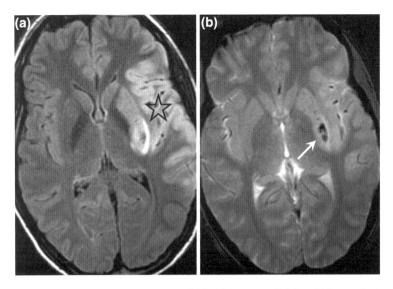

Fig. 1.1 MRI FLAIR and T2* sequences 24 h after onset of left middle cerebral artery infarction. Cerebral oedema is hyperintense on the FLAIR sequence (**a** *star*). Deep focal haemorrhagic transformation is visible as a hypointense zone on T2* images **b** *arrow*

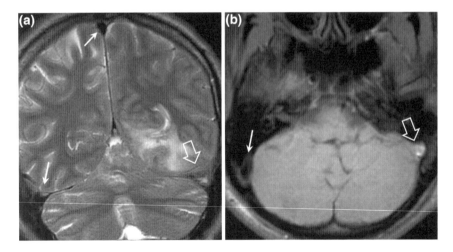

Fig. 1.2 MRI T2 and T1- weighted SE sequences in a female patient with cerebral venous thrombosis. Normal venous blood flow is hypointense on both sequences (**a** and **b** *single arrows*). Absence of venous blood flow in the thrombosed left sigmoid sinus with a hypointense signal on both sequences (**a** and **b** *hollow arrows*)

while arterial occlusion gives an iso-intense or hyperintense signal (particularly useful for middle cerebral arteries).

Fig. 1.3 Intracranial MR angiography, TOF sequence in a female patient with left middle cerebral artery infarction. Arterial blood flow in the left middle cerebral artery is interrupted by endoluminal thrombus (*hollow arrow*)

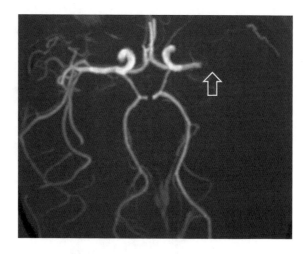

TOF or Time of Flight (Fig. 1.3)

TOF is an unenhanced T1-weighted angiography sequence. The vascular signal is favoured over that of surrounding tissues. The tissue signal is saturated and the blood flow signal entering the volume of interest is not saturated, thereby allowing reconstruction of the vessels.

Gadolinium-Enhanced MR Angiography (Fig. 1.4)

Time-of-flight sequences may present artifacts due to slow or turbulent flow, which is why it is preferable to use contrast-enhanced T1-weighted volume-rendering sequences to explore neck vessels. Signal acquisition is performed during the first pass of the contrast agent bolus in the vessels explored. The contrast agent decreases the T1 relaxation time by a factor of 10, allowing a short repetition time and rapid volume acquisition for three-dimensional reconstructions.

Diffusion-Weighted Imaging

Diffusion-weighted MRI allows exploration of random micro-movements of extracellular water molecules in a medium (Fig. 1.5). These movements depend on the obstacles encountered by water molecules in the medium. In the body, these obstacles essentially consist of proteins, cellular debris or nerve fibres. Free diffusion is said to be isotropic, i.e. water molecules diffuse freely in all directions in a pure medium such as CSF (Fig. 1.6). Isotropic diffusion can be restricted by the

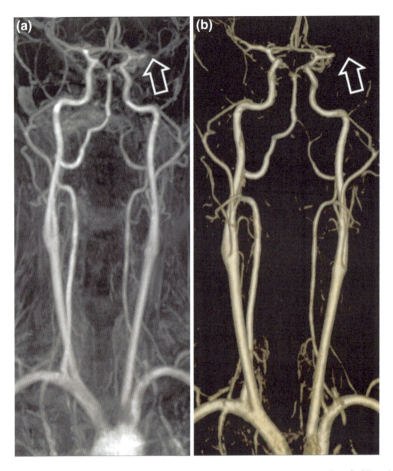

Fig. 1.4 Gadolinium-enhanced cerebral MR angiography (**a** MIP reconstruction, **b** 3D volume reconstruction) in a female patient with left middle cerebral artery infarction. Arterial blood flow in the left middle cerebral artery is interrupted by endoluminal thrombus (*hollow arrows*)

presence of an obstacle (protein or cells, etc.), as in the case of an abscess (Fig. 1.7) or a highly cellular lesion (lymphoma) (Fig. 1.8). Finally, diffusion can be anisotropic, for example when water molecules diffuse along nerve fibres (Fig. 1.9). In that case, water molecules no longer move freely in all directions, but preferably diffuse in the direction of the nerve fibres with more limited diffusion in the direction perpendicular to the nerve fibres.

Diffusion-weighted imaging depends on the attenuation factor of the b-value (s/mm^2). A b-value of 1,000 s/mm^2 is used to quantify cerebral ischaemia. The diagnostic sensitivity of diffusion-weighted imaging to detect infarction within the six first hours is 90 %.

In diffusion-weighted imaging, signal intensity depends on diffusion of water molecules, but also the prolonged T2 relaxation time. A hyperintense signal on

Fig. 1.5 Normal free isotropic diffusion. Water molecules move randomly in all directions

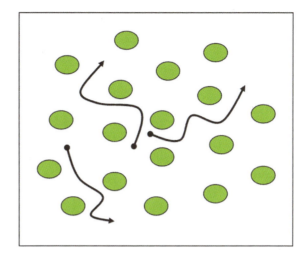

Fig. 1.6 Fluid without cellular debris: increased isotropic diffusion (cyst, tumour necrosis, CSF)

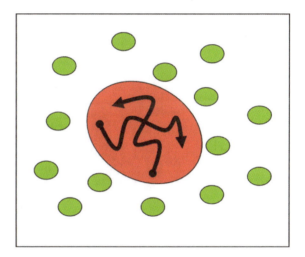

diffusion-weighted imaging can therefore be linked to a T2 effect (T2 hyperintensity) and/or increased diffusion, which is why mapping with diffusion-weighted imaging comprises T2 mapping acquisition with $b = 0$, corresponding to apparent diffusion coefficient (ADC) mapping free of T2 effects.

Increased diffusion of water molecules results in a hypointense signal on diffusion-weighted sequences and a hyperintense signal (or red on colour map) on ADC mapping (for example, CSF of ventricles). Restricted diffusion of water molecules results in a hyperintense signal on the diffusion-weighted sequence and a hypointense signal (or blue on colour map) on ADC mapping (for example, acute phase of ischaemic stroke) (Fig. 1.10).

Fig. 1.7 Fluid with cellular debris: decreased isotropic diffusion due to debris (abscess)

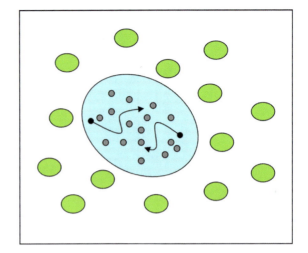

Fig. 1.8 Hypercellularity: decreased isotropic diffusion due to reduction of the extracellular space as a result of increased cellular density (e.g.: lymphoma)

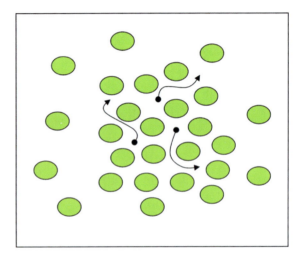

Diffusion is increased when the extracellular water volume is increased: vasogenic oedema (Fig. 1.11).

Diffusion is decreased when the extracellular water volume is decreased: cytotoxic oedema (Fig. 1.12).

- Decreased extracellular water = decreased diffusion (hyperintense on diffusion-weighted imaging):

  - increased volume of each cell = cytotoxic oedema = arterial infarction (acute phase).
  - increased number of cells (hypercellularity) = tumours (lymphoma ++), multiple sclerosis (MS) plaque.
  - decreased extracellular viscosity = abscess.

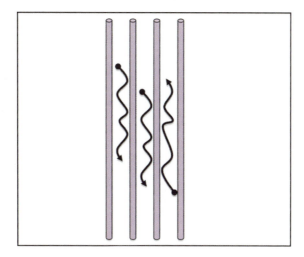

Fig. 1.9 Bundle of nerve fibres: anisotropic diffusion preferentially in the direction of the fibres (normal white matter)

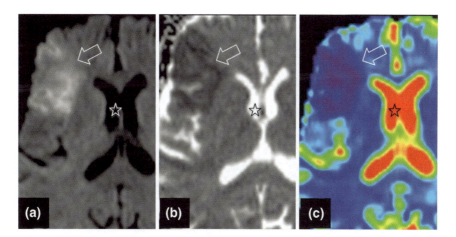

Fig. 1.10 Infarction on diffusion-weighted imaging (**a**) and black and white (**b**) and colour (**c**) ADC mapping. Pure fluids such as CSF of lateral ventricles (*star*) have increased diffusion—hypointense on diffusion-weighted images, *white* (*black and white map*) or red (*colour map*) on ADC maps. In contrast, in the case of cytotoxic oedema, such as the acute phase of infarction (*hollow arrow*), diffusion is reduced (hypointense on diffusion-weighted images), black (*black and white map*) or blue (*colour map*) on ADC maps

- Increased extracellular water = increased diffusion (hypointense on diffusion-weighted imaging):
  - decreased number of cells = gliosis.
  - increased extracellular volume = vasogenic oedema = arterial infarction (chronic phase) or venous infarction (acute and chronic phases).

Fig. 1.11 Vasogenic oedema: increased isotropic diffusion due to increased extracellular space related to extracellular oedema (arterial thrombosis [subacute or chronic phase], venous thrombosis [all phases], white matter rarefaction [gliosis])

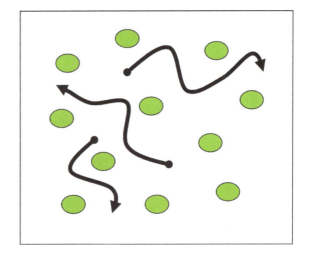

Fig. 1.12 Cytotoxic oedema: decreased isotropic diffusion due to reduction of the extracellular space related to cellular oedema (e.g.: acute phase of arterial thrombosis)

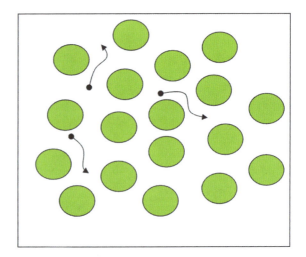

Perfusion-Weighted Imaging (Fig. 1.13)

Perfusion-weighted imaging can be used to study capillary blood flow. Perfusion may be qualitative: the pathological area is compared to a healthy area (giving a relative value) or quantitative: calibration by arrival of contrast agent in the arteries (arterial input function) or by flushing of contrast agent from the veins (venous output function).

First-pass method: injection of a contrast agent bolus and recording of the signal drop related to the T2 effect by rapid echo-planar T2 sequence or EPI *(Echo Planar Imaging)*.

Fig. 1.13 First-pass perfusion-weighted imaging, T2-weighted sequence. At t0, arrival of the contrast agent bolus is responsible for a sudden signal drop (T2 effect)

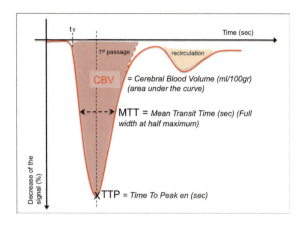

The area under the curve obtained corresponds to the cerebral blood volume (CBV). Full width at half maximum of the curve corresponds to the mean transit time (MTT). The CBV/MTT ratio corresponds to cerebral blood flow (CBF). The time to peak (TTP) corresponds to the time between the start of contrast agent injection and the peak of the curve. These parameters can be used to study the microcirculation (in the tissues), rather than blood flow in the large carotid or vertebrobasilar vessels.

CBF is expressed in mL/100 g of tissue/minute. The normal value of CBF in grey matter ranges between 50 and 60 mL/100 g/min. CBV is expressed in mL/100 g of tissue. MTT and TTP are expressed in seconds. In practice, relative values, i.e. rCBV, rCBF and rMTT, are essentially used in comparison with the healthy side (pathological side/healthy side). Colour maps are also very useful to estimate the infarcted zone and look for a penumbra zone.

Ischaemic Penumbra or Diffusion-Perfusion Mismatch (Fig. 1.14)

The ischaemic penumbra corresponds to a non-necrotic hypoperfused zone around the infarct during the acute phase. Very early thrombolysis can theoretically help to prevent or limit progression of the penumbra zone towards infarction by increasing the perfusion pressure. The penumbra zone can be fairly accurately estimated by comparing perfusion and diffusion maps. The penumbra or mismatch zone therefore corresponds to the hypoperfused zone (CBV, CBF or MTT map) characterized by decreased CBV and CBF and increased MTT, while no abnormality is yet visible on diffusion-weighted imaging (ADC map).

Note that diffusion-perfusion mismatch is different from clinico-radiological mismatch, which corresponds to discordance between the limited extent of abnormalities on diffusion-weighted imaging and the severity of clinical signs.

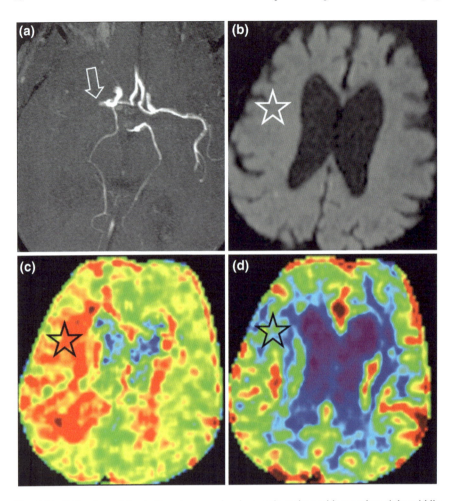

Fig. 1.14 Estimation of the ischaemic penumbra in a male patient with complete right middle cerebral artery infarction (left-sided hemiplegia) at the acute phase (first hour). On MRI, the right middle cerebral artery is amputated on the TOF sequence (**a** *hollow arrow*), with no visible abnormality in the ischaemic territory on diffusion-weighted imaging (**b** *star*). However, perfusion-weighted imaging reveals extensive abnormalities in the hypoperfused territory, with increased MTT (**c** *star*) and decreased CBV (**d** *star*). The penumbra or mismatch involves all of the right middle cerebral artery territory that is hypoperfused, but not yet ischaemic at the early stage at which the examination was performed due to collateral circulation. This situation is inevitably temporary: the penumbra may resolve if perfusion pressure is increased (for example by early revascularization of the occluded artery) with no subsequent infarction, or, on the contrary, the penumbra may progress to infarction if perfusion pressure remains low in the absence of early revascularization and/or a fall in blood pressure

MRI Contraindications

- Claustrophobic patient.
- Patient with a mechanical heart valve or pacemaker.
- Intraorbital metallic foreign body.
- Cochlear implants.
- Severe obesity (>140/150 kg).
- Ferromagnetic vascular clips.

Precautions for Imaging Procedures (CT and MRI)

(CIRTACI guidelines (*Comité interdisciplinaire de recherche et de travail sur les agents de contraste en imagerie*—SFR multidisciplinary contrast agent task force).

Pregnancy

As a precaution, any non-urgent examination other than ultrasound that can be performed after delivery must be deferred until after delivery.

Due to the insufficient data available in pregnant women, injection of an MRI contrast agent is not recommended, but can be performed after careful assessment of the risk/benefit balance.

When imaging is formally indicated and when injection of an MRI contrast agent is essential, the examination can be performed at any time during pregnancy.

When an iodinated contrast agent is used after 12 weeks of amenorrhoea, the paediatric team must be informed to ensure monitoring of the newborn child's thyroid function, as this brief iodine overload can induce transient foetal thyroid dysfunction.

Renal Insufficiency

Iodine

Impaired renal function can occur during the 72 h following injection of an iodinated contrast agent. This contrast agent-induced nephropathy is defined by elevation of baseline serum creatinine by more than 42 μmol/L and/or more than 25 %.

Risk factors

- Pre-existing renal insufficiency: creatinine clearance <60 mL/min.
- Diabetes with renal insufficiency.

- Renal hypoperfusion.
- Use of nephrotoxic drugs.
- Multiple myeloma with proteinuria.
- Injection of iodinated contrast agents during the previous 3 days.
- Age >65 years.

Precautions

- A minimum interval of 3 days and preferably 5 days must be observed between 2 successive injections of iodinated contrast agent.
- Good hydration of the patient.
- Use of low-osmolality or iso-osmolality contrast agents in patients with risk factors.
- Treatment with metformin derivatives must be stopped for 48 h after the contrast agent injection (treatment does not need to be stopped 48 h before the injection). Treatment is resumed after confirming the absence of impaired renal function.

Gadolinium

Cases of nephrogenic systemic fibrosis have been reported in patients with severe renal insufficiency following gadolinium injection, particularly with gadodiamide (Omniscan®). This is a rare complication with extensive cutaneous and sometimes deep tissue fibrosis, mostly affecting the limbs.

Precautions

- Creatinine clearance <30 mL/min or candidate for renal transplantation: Omniscan® is contraindicated. Use other gadolinium contrast agents after assessing the risk/benefit balance.
- Creatinine clearance between 30 and 60 mL/min: no particular recommendation.

Chapter 2
General Description of Cerebral Infarction

Vascular Anatomy of Cerebral Arteries

The cerebral blood supply is derived from four neck vessels: 2 internal carotid arteries (Fig. 2.1) and 2 vertebral arteries (Fig. 2.2). The vertebral arteries merge in the midline to form the basilar artery.

Inside the skull, each internal carotid artery bifurcates to form the anterior cerebral artery and the middle cerebral artery. The basilar artery gives rise to two posterior cerebral arteries.

The anterior system, composed of 2 internal carotid arteries, and the posterior system composed of the vertebrobasilar system, communicate in the Circle of Willis (Fig. 2.3) via communicating arteries: an anterior communicating artery and two posterior communicating arteries. The anterior communicating artery connects the 2 anterior cerebral arteries in the midline. The posterior communicating artery connects the internal carotid artery to the ipsilateral posterior cerebral artery.

The cerebral blood supply (Fig. 2.4) is ensured by the anterior, middle and posterior cerebral arteries but also by the anterior choroidal artery derived from the posterior aspect of the terminal internal carotid artery and perforating vessels derived from the posterior communicating arteries.

The blood supply of the brainstem and cerebellum (Fig. 2.5) is ensured by arteries derived from the terminal vertebral arteries (namely posterior inferior cerebellar artery or PICA and perforating branches) and arteries derived from the basilar artery (anterior inferior cerebellar arteries or AICA, superior cerebellar and perforating vessel system).

Arterial Anatomical Variants

Many anatomical variants of intracranial or extracranial arteries to the brain can be observed. The internal carotid arteries present the same diameter on each side, while the vertebral arteries are often asymmetrical.

G. Saliou et al., *Practical Guide to Neurovascular Emergencies*,
DOI: 10.1007/978-2-8178-0481-1_2, © Springer-Verlag France 2014

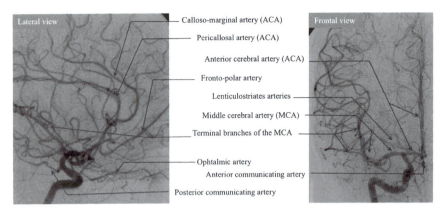

Fig. 2.1 Angiographic anatomy of the right internal carotid artery

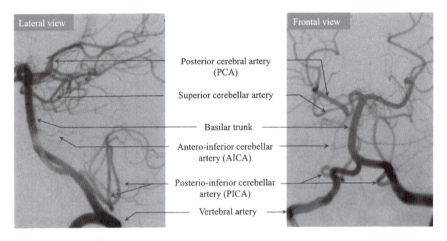

Fig. 2.2 Angiographic anatomy of the vertebrobasilar system

Fig. 2.3 Diagram of the Circle of Willis (*inferior view*). *ACA* anterior cerebral artery, *MCA* middle cerebral artery, *PCA* posterior cerebral artery, *IC* internal carotid artery, *BT* basilar trunk, *A*-Com anterior communicating artery, *P*-Com posterior communicating artery

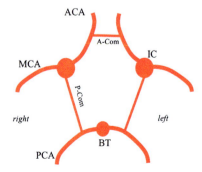

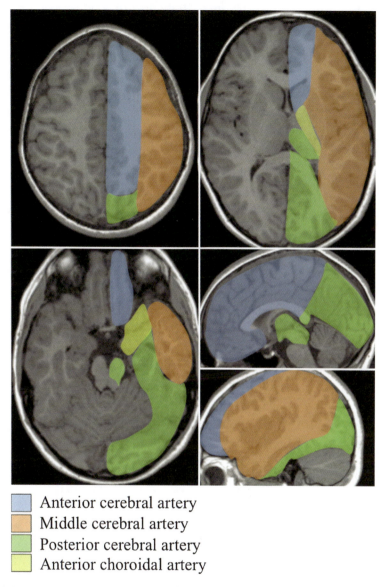

■ Anterior cerebral artery
■ Middle cerebral artery
■ Posterior cerebral artery
■ Anterior choroidal artery

Fig. 2.4 Vascular territories of the brain

In the presence of asymmetrical internal carotid arteries (Fig. 2.6), the size of the petrous and cavernous portions of the carotid canal must be studied first.

A small carotid canal on the side of the narrowed internal carotid artery corresponds to very rare constitutional asymmetry. Otherwise, this asymmetry may indicate secondary internal carotid artery stenosis (dissection, atherosclerosis, cerebral vasculitis, etc.)

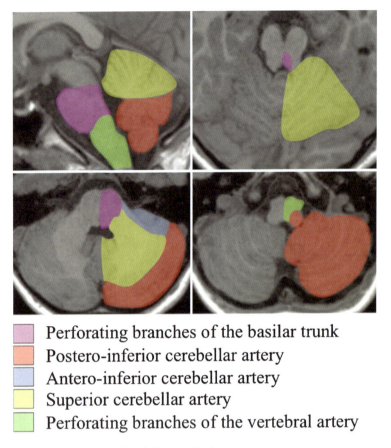

◻ Perforating branches of the basilar trunk
◻ Postero-inferior cerebellar artery
◻ Antero-inferior cerebellar artery
◻ Superior cerebellar artery
◻ Perforating branches of the vertebral artery

Fig. 2.5 Vascular territories of cerebellum and brainstem

The vertebral arteries are often asymmetrical, with about 40 % of vertebral arteries of equal size, a dominant left vertebral artery in 35–40 % of cases, and a dominant right vertebral artery in 20–25 % of cases (Fig. 2.7). Marked hypoplasia is observed in 9 % of cases for the right vertebral artery and nearly 6 % of cases for the left vertebral artery. Bilateral hypoplasia of the vertebral arteries is described in 0.75 % of cases. In constitutional asymmetry, the size of the artery remains regular over its entire length with a terminal V4 segment also smaller than the contralateral V4 segment. The diameter of the V4 segment of artery can also be smaller after the origin of the PICA and in case of hypoplasia of the V4 segment. The vertebral artery may even terminate in the posterior inferior cerebellar artery (PICA) on the side of the small vertebral artery.

Many anatomical variants of the Circle of Willis have been described. The most common variants are a 'foetal' disposition of the posterior cerebral artery, which arises directly from the internal carotid artery via the posterior communicating artery, and hypoplasia of the first segment of the anterior cerebral artery (A1 segment),

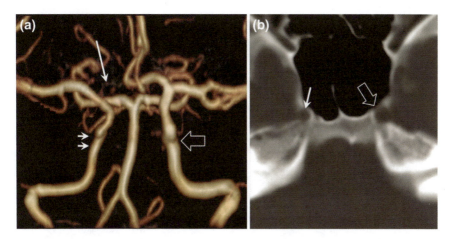

Fig. 2.6 Constitutional asymmetry of internal carotid arteries with a hypoplastic right carotid artery (**a** intracranial MR angiography, *anterior view*; *double arrows*: right internal carotid artery, *hollow arrow*: left internal carotid artery). CT confirms the presence of a constitutional variant by demonstrating a small carotid canal on the side of the hypoplastic right internal carotid artery (**b** *single arrow*) compared with the left carotid canal (**b** *hollow arrow*). Also note another variant in this patient with hypoplasia of the first segment of the right anterior cerebral artery (**a** *arrow*); both anterior cerebral arteries are supplied by the left internal carotid artery

in which the artery arises directly from the contralateral internal carotid artery via the anterior communicating artery (Fig. 2.8). These anatomical variants can explain why infarction due to occlusion of a neck artery can extend to adjacent arterial territories and wrongly suggest a cardioembolic origin (Fig. 2.9).

Anatomy of Cerebral Veins

The cerebral venous system presents a wide range of anatomical variants.

Nevertheless, three distinct cerebral venous systems communicating with each other can be identified: deep and superficial venous system and cavernous sinus. The deep and superficial venous systems communicate with each other via the confluence of sinuses or torcular.

The superficial venous system (Fig. 2.10) includes the superior sagittal sinus, which drains into the torcular posteriorly. The superior sagittal sinus receives numerous cortical veins, the largest of which is the superior anastomotic vein (vein of Trolard). Blood from the torcular is drained by the left and right transverse sinuses and the sigmoid sinuses and finally the internal jugular veins that leave the skull via the jugular foramina. Several cortical veins drain into the sigmoid sinuses and transverse sinuses, the largest of which is the inferior anastomotic vein (vein of Labbé).

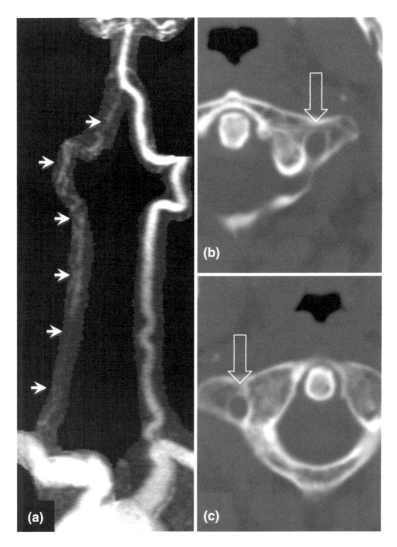

Fig. 2.7 Cerebral MR angiography showing classical features of constitutional asymmetry of the vertebral arteries with a dominant left vertebral artery and a hypoplastic right vertebral artery (**a** *arrows*). Note that the transverse foramina are not asymmetrical despite the difference in size of the arteries due to the numerous venous plexuses that also travel along the course of the vertebral arteries (**b** cervical spine CT scan, *hollow arrow*, left transverse foramen; **c** *hollow arrow*, right transverse foramen)

The deep venous system (Fig. 2.11) comprises the midline inferior sagittal sinus, the paramedian deep cerebral veins and the basal veins around the midbrain. All of these veins converge posteriorly to form the great cerebral vein of Galien that drains into the straight sinus and finally the torcular, where the deep and superficial systems meet. The basal veins also drain anteriorly into the cavernous sinus.

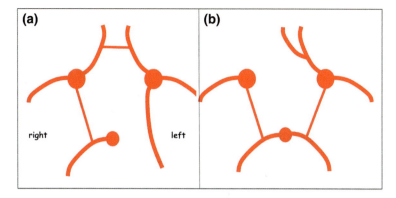

Fig. 2.8 Diagrams of the Circle of Willis (*inferior view*). Examples of anatomical variants with foetal disposition of the left posterior cerebral artery (**a**) arising directly from the posterior communicating artery. The first P1 segment is generally present but hypoplastic. Another classical variant (**b**) with hypoplasia of the first segment of the right anterior cerebral artery. In this case, both anterior cerebral arteries arise from the same internal carotid artery and have a common first segment

The cavernous sinus is a pericarotid venous network situated laterally to the body of the sphenoid. It drains the majority of facial veins and part of the deep cerebral venous system via the basal veins and superficial cortical veins via the superficial middle cerebral veins.

Epidemiology of Cerebral Infarction

Leading cause of acquired disability in adults.
Second leading cause of dementia (after Alzheimer's disease).
Third leading cause of death.
20 % mortality at 1 month; 1/3 of survivors are dependent for activities of daily living.

Incidence
Ranging from 210 to 600/100,000 inhabitants per year, according to the country.

One-year recurrence rate without treatment

- 12 % for cardioembolic infarcts.
- 15 % for infarcts due to atherosclerotic carotid artery stenosis when not operated.

One-Year Recurrence Rate with Treatment

- 2 % for atrial fibrillation (AF) treated by oral anticoagulants.
- 3 % for carotid artery infarction after surgical treatment of atherosclerotic carotid artery stenosis.

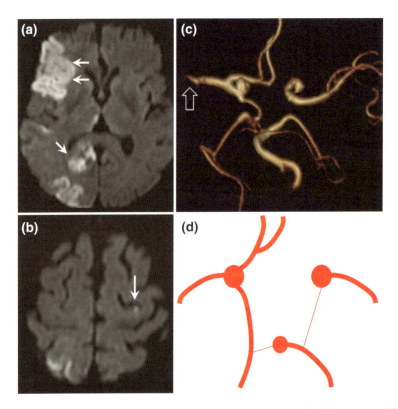

Fig. 2.9 Patient with infarction in 3 distinct territories: right MCA (**a** *double arrow*) and PCA (**a** *single arrow*) territories and distal left ACA territory (**b** *arrow*). Infarction is due to emboli derived from the right internal carotid artery. Anatomical variants of the Circle of Willis in this patient account for infarction in these 3 territories: common origin of the 2 anterior cerebral arteries from the right internal carotid artery (hypoplasia of first segment of the left internal carotid artery) and foetal disposition of the right posterior cerebral artery arising directly from the right posterior communicating artery (**c** MR angiography with 3D reconstruction, *inferior view*); **d** diagram showing the variants in this patient. The right middle cerebral artery is interrupted by an embolus (**c** *hollow arrow*)

Risk Factors

- Non-modifiable: age, male gender (incidence 1.25 × female gender).
- Modifiable: hypertension (risk × 4), dyslipidaemia (risk × 1.5), smoking (risk × 1.5), diabetes (risk × 3), alcohol (risk × 3–6), obesity (risk × 2), oral contraceptive (risk × 2), AF (leading cause of cardioembolic stroke and 50 % of cardioembolic strokes in rich countries).

Fig. 2.10 Lateral view
(**a**) and oblique view (**b**) of
the superficial cerebral
venous system. *1* Superior
sagittal sinus. *2* Torcular. *3*
Straight sinus (sectioned). *4*
Transverse sinus. *5* Sigmoid
sinus. *6* Inferior anastomotic
veins (veins of Labbé). *7*
Superior anastomotic veins
(veins of Trolard)

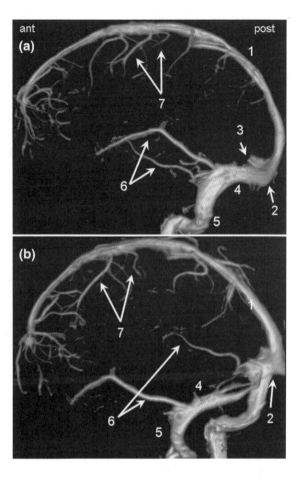

Imaging of Acute Cerebral Infarction

CT

CT generally visualizes signs of ischaemia by the third hour (Fig. 2.12).
   These signs vary according to the territory concerned:

– Middle cerebral artery: **loss of the normal contour of the basal ganglia**
   compared with the contralateral side and **loss of the cortical sulci** of the lateral
   sulcus due to oedema.
– Anterior and posterior cerebral arteries and superficial territory of the middle
   cerebral artery: loss of **cortical-subcortical differentiation**, cortical grey matter
   becomes hypodense, blurring with the adjacent white matter.

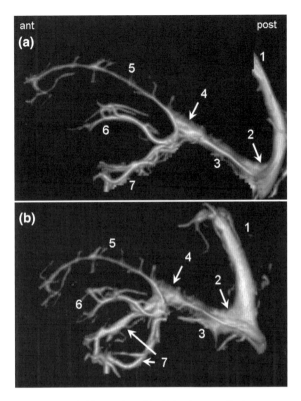

Fig. 2.11 Lateral view (**a**) and oblique view (**b**) of the deep cerebral venous system. *1* Superior sagittal sinus (sectioned). *2* Torcular. *3* Straight sinus. *4* Great cerebral vein of Galien. *5* Inferior sagittal sinus. *6* Deep cerebral veins. *7* Basal veins (of Rosenthal)

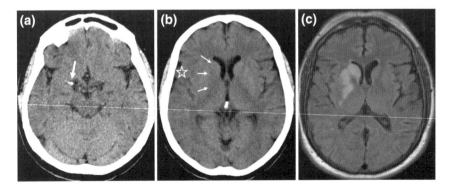

Fig. 2.12 Early signs of deep middle cerebral artery infarction on CT scan. Hyperdensity of first segment (M1) of the right middle cerebral artery (**a** *arrow*) due to the presence of intra-arterial clot caused by thrombosis or embolism with loss of the normal contours of the basal ganglia (**b** *triple arrows*) compared with the contralateral side. Slight loss of cortical sulci of the lateral sulcus (*star*) due to oedema. MRI FLAIR sequence (**c**) confirms the hyperintense deep middle cerebral artery infarction

The clot in the artery is generally visualized at an early stage, within the first minutes, as a **linear hyperdensity**.

In the case of haemorrhagic transformation of the infarction or primary haemorrhagic stroke, bleeding is visualized as a hyperdensity within the hypo-density of the affected cerebral parenchyma.

MRI

MRI visualizes early signs of ischaemia within 30 min for morphological sequences and by the first minutes for perfusion-weighted sequences (Figs. 2.13 and 2.14).

- Restricted diffusion (hyperintensity) with early decrease of ADC by 30 min. ADC then gradually returns to normal after about 10 days, and subsequently increases thereafter (Fig. 2.15).
- FLAIR and T2-weighted imaging: hyperintensity of ischaemic parenchyma by the third hour.
- Perfusion-weighted imaging: abnormalities are visible at an early stage, by the first minutes, as decreased cerebral blood volume (CBV) and cerebral blood flow (CBF) and increased mean transit time (MTT).
- On T2-weighted gradient-echo imaging, the clot may be visible in the artery as endoluminal hypointensity.
- On TOF sequences: arterial occlusion or stenosis. N.B.: TOF sequences are T1-weighted and the occlusive intravascular clot may appear spontaneously hyperintense on T1-weighted imaging, giving a falsely patent appearance of the artery: carefully examine the distal run-off, which is poorer than on the healthy contralateral side.

In the case of haemorrhagic transformation of the infarction or primary haemorrhagic stroke, bleeding appears hypointense within the ischaemic zone on T2-weighted gradient-echo sequences.

Collateral Circulation (Fig. 2.16)

Following proximal occlusion of an artery, distal collateral circulation may be ensured by leptomeningeal anastomoses with distal arteries of adjacent territories. A classical example is deep middle cerebral artery infarction (lenticulostriate arteries derived from the M1 segment of the middle cerebral artery) without superficial middle cerebral artery infarction despite occlusion of the origin of the middle cerebral artery. Ischaemia is observed in the lenticulostriate territory, in which the blood supply is terminal, in contrast with the superficial territory, in which the cortical branches of the MCA can be supplied by pial anastomoses with

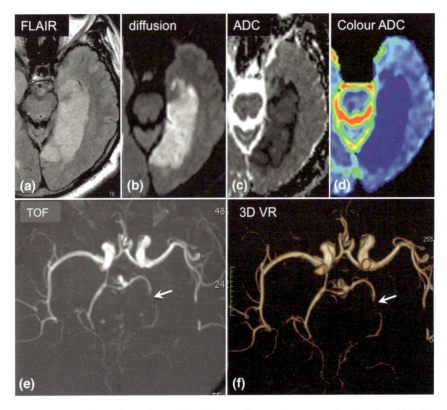

Fig. 2.13 Infarction in the territory of the left posterior cerebral artery after less than 24 h. The infarct is visible on FLAIR sequences (**a**) and diffusion-weighted imaging (**b**) as areas of hyperintensity. Apparent diffusion coefficient (ADC) mapping appears hypointense (**c**) on black and white maps or more intensely blue than the adjacent healthy parenchyma on colour maps (**d**). Arterial time-of-flight (TOF) MR angiography of the Circle of Willis (**e** *inferior view*) and 3D volume reconstruction (**f** volume rendering or VR) showing loss of the intravascular signal in the left posterior cerebral artery (*arrow*) compared to the healthy contralateral side

the ACA and/or PCA territories. This collateral circulation may subsequently be insufficient over the hours and days following onset of the symptoms, particularly in a context of poor haemodynamic conditions, such as low blood pressure or intracranial hypertension, possibly resulting in extension of deep infarction towards superficial territories, resulting in complete infarction (Fig. 2.17).

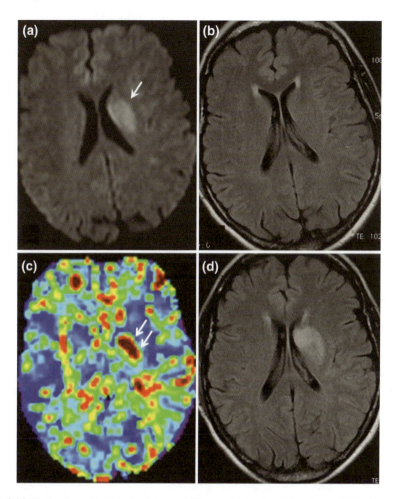

Fig. 2.14 Early phase (1st hour) of deep middle cerebral artery infarction on MRI. Note the absence of abnormalities on the FLAIR sequence (**b**) with abnormal diffusion-weighted (**a** *arrow*) and perfusion-weighted sequences (*c* markedly increased MTT, double arrows), demonstrating the cerebral ischaemia (decreased ADC and marked increase of MTT). Follow-up MRI 24 h later (**d**) shows the appearance of ischaemic abnormalities on FLAIR imaging

Clinical Signs of Cerebral Infarction

The site of infarction can often be predicted on the basis of clinical signs. However, only neuroradiological assessment can demonstrate the affected territory and the extent of infarction.

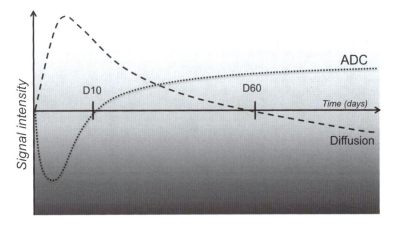

Fig. 2.15 Signal variation on diffusion-weighted imaging and ADC mapping as a function of time after onset of ischaemic stroke

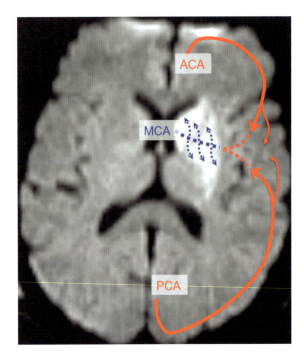

Fig. 2.16 Occlusion of the first segment (M1) of the middle cerebral artery (*MCA*) responsible for infarction (hyperintense on this diffusion-weighted sequence) of its deep territory (lenticulostriate arteries shown as *blue* on the diagram). The *MCA* no longer supplies the superficial cortical arteries. There is no infarction in the superficial middle cerebral artery territory due to the leptomeningeal collateral vessels allowing anastomosis of the superficial cortical network of the *MCA* to adjacent territories of the anterior cerebral artery (*ACA*) and posterior cerebral artery (*PCA*)

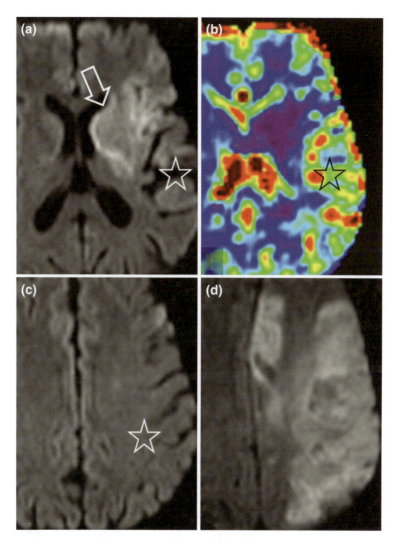

Fig. 2.17 Deep middle cerebral artery infarction (**a** diffusion-weighted sequence, *hollow arrow*) due to occlusion of the first segment of the middle cerebral artery. The superficial territory is spared due to leptomeningeal collateral vessels (**a** and **c** diffusion-weighted sequence, *star*) with no abnormality of the superficial cerebral perfusion (**b** *star*). At 24 h, secondary extension of the infarct to the superficial territory due to insufficient collateral circulation (**d** diffusion-weighted sequence)

Carotid Territory

Middle Cerebral Artery Infarction

MCA infarction is the most common form of cerebral infarction (70 % of carotid artery infarcts).

Limited MCA Infarction

- **Infarction of the deep territory of the MCA (Fig.** 2.18)

Infarction of the deep territory is due to occlusion of perforating branches, causing ischaemia of the internal capsule and basal ganglia.

- Constant contralateral motor deficit, often complete and proportional. Patients with partial motor deficit at least present motor neglect.
- Inconsistent sensory and visual field deficit (depending on the posterior and lateral extension of infarction towards the optic radiations).
- Frequent cognitive disorders: motor aphasia (left-sided lesion) or anosognosia (right-sided lesion).

Fig. 2.18 Deep middle cerebral artery infarction. Hyperintensity on diffusion-weighted imaging of the head of the caudate nucleus (*single arrow*) and lentiform nucleus (*double arrows*)

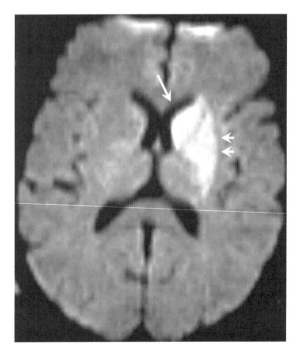

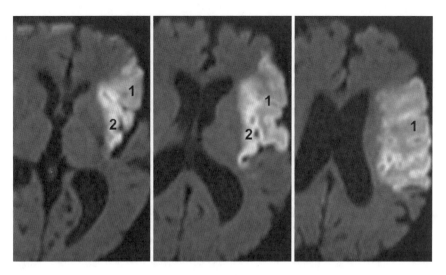

Fig. 2.19 Superficial middle cerebral artery infarction, frontal branch. Hyperintensity on diffusion-weighted imaging in the frontal cortex (*1*) and insula (*2*)

- **Infarction limited to the cortical territory of the MCA**

The clinical features are fairly typical and suggestive due to organization of the motor and sensory areas according to the homunculus.

We will confine ourselves to the main stroke syndromes observed in the context of MCA cortical infarction:

- Frontal stroke (anterior opercular syndrome (Fig. 2.19): severe brachiofacial motor deficit with impaired swallowing and mastication, Broca's aphasia (left-sided lesion) or anosognosia (right-sided lesion).
- Parietotemporal stroke (Fig. 2.20): mainly sensory deficit, predominantly brachiofacial, Wernicke's aphasia (left-sided lesion), homonymous hemianopsia (left-sided lesion), left hemifield visual deficit or visual neglect (right-sided lesion).

Total MCA Infarction (Fig. 2.21)

Twenty to 35 % of carotid artery stenoses result in total MCA infarction, responsible for severe clinical features that may be immediately life-threatening due to uncal herniation, corresponding to malignant middle cerebral artery infarction:

- Proportional hemibody motor deficit with hemianaesthesia.
- Homonymous hemianopsia.
- Conjugate deviation of the head and eyes to the side of the lesion.

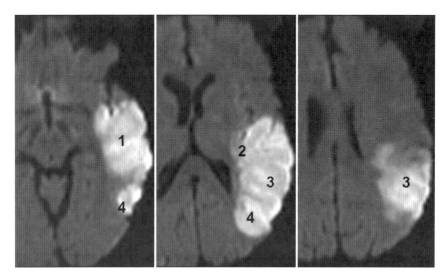

Fig. 2.20 Superficial middle cerebral artery infarction, parietotemporal branch. Hyperintensity on diffusion-weighted imaging in the temporal cortex (*1*), posterior insula (*2*), parietal cortex (*3*) and occipital cortex (*4*)

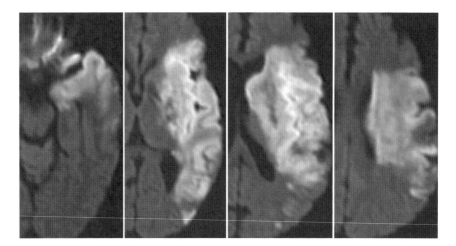

Fig. 2.21 Total middle cerebral artery infarction. Hyperintensity on diffusion-weighted imaging in the superficial and deep territories

- Impaired alertness and breathing (Cheyne-Stokes breathing).
- Cognitive disorders: global aphasia (left-sided lesion) or disorders of body awareness: hemiasomatognosia, anosognosia and left unilateral spatial neglect (right-sided lesion).
- Bilateral Babinski's sign.

Anterior cerebral artery infarction (rare) (Fig. 2.22)

- Complete infarction in the territory of the ACA
- Motor deficit, predominantly affecting the proximal muscles of the lower limbs.
- Sensory disorders with a similar distribution.
- Incontinence, generally transient.
- Frontal syndrome (grasp reflex).
- Speech disorder (initially muteness, followed by motor aphasia) if left-sided lesion).
- Mood disorders (apathy, moria).

Anterior choroidal artery infarction (Fig. 2.23)

Typical symptoms and multiple variants have been described according to the extent of ischaemia.

- Classical clinical triad:

  - contralateral motor deficit of variable severity and distribution,
  - hemianaesthesia affecting all modalities,
  - homonymous hemianopsia,

- Other possible associated symptoms:

  speech disorders (reduced verbal fluency sometimes associated with semantic paraphasia),

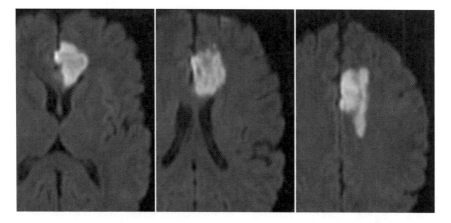

Fig. 2.22 Left ACA infarction (pericallosal artery). Hyperintensity on diffusion-weighted imaging in left pericallosal and frontal region

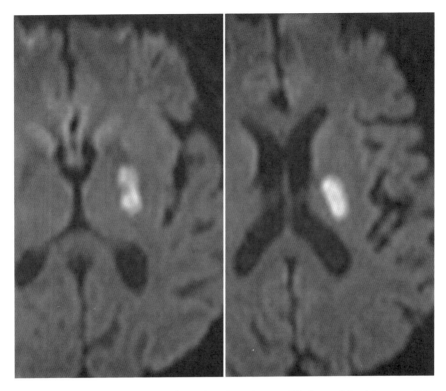

Fig. 2.23 Anterior choroidal infarction. Hyperintensity on diffusion-weighted images of the posterior limb of internal capsule. This anatomical region corresponds to passage of the pyramidal tract

neuropsychological disorders, mainly in right-sided lesions with nondominant hemisphere syndrome (neglect essentially observed during visual spatial activities),

hemiataxia (or cerebellar ataxia) ipsilateral to the motor deficit.

The clinical features can therefore mimic extensive middle cerebral artery infarction, but are rarely associated with impaired level of consciousness and conjugate deviation of the head and eyes.

Vertebrobasilar Territory

As the basilar artery is a single artery, the side of basilar artery and PCA infarctions cannot predict which vertebral artery is involved; this is not the case with posterior inferior cerebellar artery infarctions (as the PICA arises from the ipsilateral vertebral artery). Brainstem infarctions are usually due to stenosis or occlusion of perforating vessels of the basilar artery.

Posterior Cerebral Artery Infarction

The posterior cerebral artery is the second most common site of cerebral infarction.

Infarction of the Superficial Territory of the PCA (Fig. 2.24)

The clinical features are dominated by simple or complex visual disorders:

- contralateral homonymous hemianopsia,
- visual hallucinations, metamorphopsia (distorted vision),
- motion blindness and loss of 3D vision,
- alexia, Wernicke's aphasia if left-sided lesion,
- loss of spatial orientation, prosopagnosia (face blindness), visual hemineglect (if right-sided lesion),
- in the case of bilateral involvement: double hemianopsia, cortical blindness, visual agnosia, prosopagnosia.

Infarction of the Deep Territory of the PCA (Fig. 2.25)

These strokes comprise hemiparesis secondary to a mesencephalic lesion and a thalamic syndrome. Blood supply to the thalamus is mainly derived from the vertebrobasilar system, apart from the tuberothalamic territory which is supplied by the posterior communicating artery and therefore depends on both the carotid system and the vertebrobasilar system. Apart from posterior choroidal artery infarction (pulvinar, geniculate body), mainly causing visual disorders (homonymous quadranopsia), thalamic lesions are characterized by hemibody sensory impairment affecting all modalities, including the face, contralateral to the lesion.

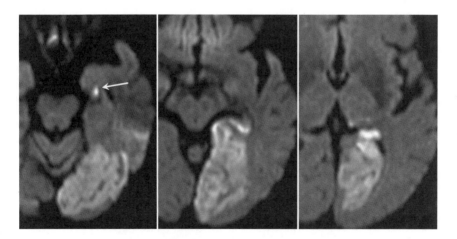

Fig. 2.24 Infarction of the superficial territory of the posterior cerebral artery. Hyperintensity on diffusion-weighted images predominantly in the medial occipital region and extending over the medial aspect of the temporal lobe (*arrow*)

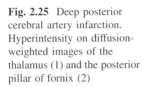
Fig. 2.25 Deep posterior cerebral artery infarction. Hyperintensity on diffusion-weighted images of the thalamus (1) and the posterior pillar of fornix (2)

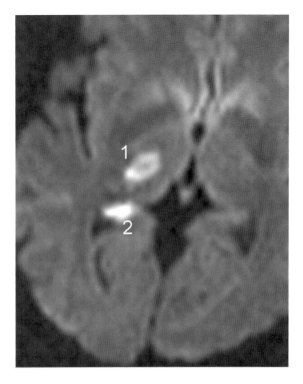

The thalamus is the major relay for all sensory modalities, **hence the risk of secondary thalamic pain syndrome**.

Other features of thalamic syndromes

- Tuberothalamic territory:

    – aphasia, amnesia, if lesion is left-sided,
    – visuospatial hemineglect if lesion is right-sided,
    – moderate hemiparesis.

- Paramedian territory: often bilateral involvement as these regions are supplied by a single pedicle (Fig. 2.26):

    – disorders of consciousness, hypersomnia,
    – vertical gaze palsy, bilateral ptosis,
    – memory disorders,
    – athymhormia.

Extensive PCA Infarction (Fig. 2.27)

The clinical presentation can mimic MCA or anterior choroidal artery occlusion, combining:

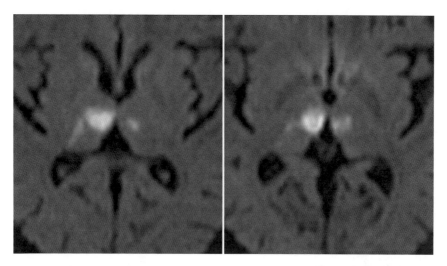

Fig. 2.26 Terminal basilar artery infarction. Bithalamic hyperintensity on diffusion-weighted imaging This ischaemic stroke is bilateral due to occlusion of all perforating arteries arising from the terminal segment of the basilar artery and the origin of the PCAs or due to occlusion of an anatomical variant, the artery of Percheron. This solitary artery arises from the termination of the basilar artery in the midline and gives rise to bilateral thalamic arteries

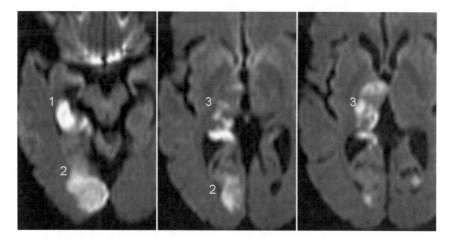

Fig. 2.27 Complete posterior cerebral artery infarction. Hyperintensity on diffusion-weighted images of the medial temporal (1) and medial occipital (2) regions and the thalamus (3)

- hemiplegia (midbrain lesion),
- hemihypesthesia (thalamic lesion),
- homonymous hemianopsia (occipital lesion).

Posterior Fossa (Brainstem and Cerebellum) Infarction

These strokes are usually due to small-vessel disease (lacunar infarcts) or basilar (pons, midbrain) or vertebral atherosclerosis (medulla oblongata) and are responsible for very varied clinical presentations.

Basilar Artery Territory (Figs. 2.28 and 2.29)

Classical "alternate hemiplegia syndrome" defined by peripheral lesion of a cranial nerve ipsilateral to the infarct (due to a lesion of the cranial nerve nucleus) and a lesion of the contralateral long tracts (sensory or motor). In practice, pure alternate hemiplegia syndromes as historically described (Weber's, Foville's, Benedikt's syndromes) are exceptional. A peripheral lesion of one or more cranial nerves (especially the oculomotor nerves) in a context of a central hemiparesis or tetraparesis is highly suggestive of brainstem stroke, a particularly important sign

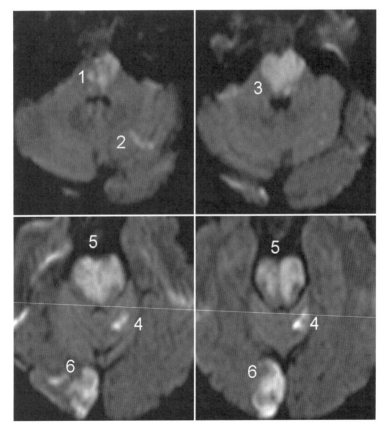

Fig. 2.28 Extensive posterior fossa infarction due to basilar artery thrombosis. Hyperintensity on diffusion-weighted imaging of the medulla oblongata (1) and left cerebellum (2), pons (3), left vermis (4), midbrain (5) and right occipital lobe (6)

Fig. 2.29 Left paramedian pontine infarction (territory of the perforating branches of the basilar artery). Hyperintensity on diffusion-weighted images of the left part of the pons

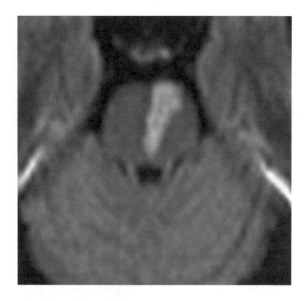

as this region is poorly visible on CT and such lesions always require confirmation by MRI.

The most serious complication of brainstem stroke or TIA is locked-in syndrome caused by bilateral paramedian pontine infarction .

Locked-in syndrome is a very severe condition combining tetraplegia, bilateral abducens and facial nerve palsy and mutism. Level of consciousness and cognitive functions remain normal. Only vertical gaze is preserved (as described in the book and the movie 'The Diving bell and the Butterfly').

Anterior Inferior Cerebellar Artery (AICA) Territory (Fig. 2.30)

Vertigo, sometimes isolated, cerebellar postural instability, involvement of ipsilateral trigeminal, facial and vestibulocochlear nerves, contralateral hemihypesthesia for pain and temperature, isolated vestibular syndrome.

Superior Cerebellar Artery Territory

Ipsilateral cerebellar ataxia, contralateral hemihypesthesia for pain and temperature and involvement of contralateral trochlear nerve, cerebellar dysarthria, nystagmus.

Vertebral Artery Territory

- Lateral medullary infarction (territory of the artery to the lateral part of medulla oblongata) (the most common form of brainstem infarction).
  Wallenberg's syndrome, comprising (Fig. 2.31):

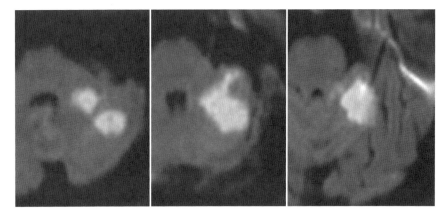

Fig. 2.30 Left AICA (anterior inferior cerebellar artery) infarction. Left cerebellar hyperintensity on diffusion-weighted imaging

Fig. 2.31 Left lateral medullary infarction (territory of the perforating branches of the basilar artery). Hyperintensity on diffusion-weighted images of the left lateral part of the medulla oblongata

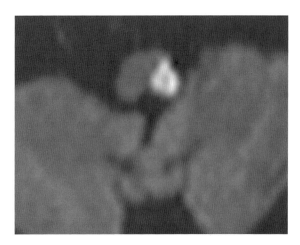

- *Ipsilateral* sensory disorders of the face (trigeminal nerve territory), Horner's syndrome (ptosis, miosis, enophthalmos), facial, glossopharyngeal and vagus nerve palsy, vestibular syndrome, cerebellar ataxia, .
- *Contralateral* hemibody sensory disorders (pain and temperature), excluding the face.

- Medial medullary infarction:

  - Ipsilateral hypoglossal nerve palsy, hemiplegia and contralateral hemihypesthesia excluding the face and rotational or spontaneous vertical nystagmus.

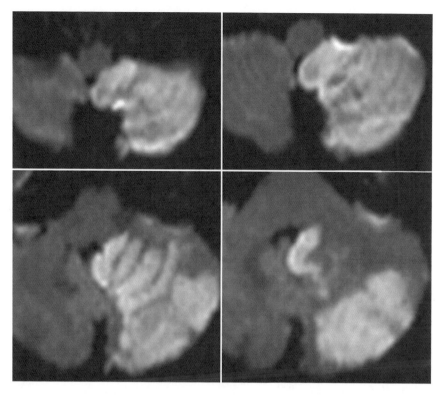

Fig. 2.32 Left PICA (posterior inferior cerebellar artery) infarction. Left cerebellar hyperintensity on diffusion-weighted images

- Cerebellar stroke:
  - Posterior inferior cerebellar artery infarction (Fig. 2.32).
  - The most common form of cerebellar stroke, generally related to vertebral artery atherosclerosis.
  - Vertigo, sometimes isolated, ipsilateral cerebellar ataxia and postural instability, dysarthria.
  - Cerebellar strokes due to PICA occlusion can sometimes be extensive (particularly in the presence of AICA aplasia) and can sometimes be life-threatening (oedema around the lesion with tonsillar herniation and/or compression of the 4th ventricle with acute non-communicating hydrocephalus).

Outcome of Cerebral Infarction

Early Outcome of Territory Infarction

Haemorrhagic Transformation (Fig. 2.33)

Definition

Haemorrhagic transformation of an ischaemic infarct is essentially due to disruption of the blood-brain barrier (BBB) and reperfusion.

It has a variable onset, from 24 to 48 h and up to 3 weeks after infarction.

Two types of haemorrhagic transformation are observed: haemorrhagic infarction (confluent or nonconfluent petechial haemorrhages in the infarcted territory: 62 % of cases) or intra-infarct haematoma (haemorrhagic collection in the infarcted territory with mass effect on adjacent structures: 37 % of cases). Haemorrhagic transformation is a factor of poor prognosis, particularly in the case of haematoma.

Petechial haemorrhage may be asymptomatic.

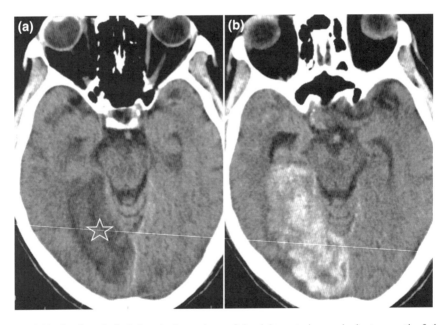

Fig. 2.33 Cardioembolic infarct in the territory of the right posterior cerebral artery on the 3rd day (**a** *star*) and the 15th day (**b**) on scan. Extensive haemorrhagic transformation on the 15th day with worsening of clinical symptoms and appearance of hyperdensity in all of the infarcted territory

Epidemiology

Radiological diagnosis is variable depending on the time of onset, the size and the cause of the infarction: 2.2–40 %. 8.7 % of cases of haemorrhagic transformation occur during the first five days.

Risk Factors

- Advanced age.
- Thrombolytic, anticoagulant and, more rarely, antiplatelet treatments.
- Pre-existing white matter disease (hyperintensity on FLAIR and T2 imaging).
- Extensive infarction.
- Early disruption of the BBB.
- Thrombolysis protocol violation.
- Cardioembolic origin: more than one half of haemorrhagic transformations are due to cardioembolic infarctions; this risk is twofold higher than after athero-sclerotic infarction with a variable incidence according to the studies: 17 % in the first week, 25–50 % after 3 weeks.

Treatment

No specific treatment. Depending on the severity of bleeding, its site and the potential risk of life-threatening uncal herniation (cerebellar infarct, for example), temporary discontinuation of antithrombotic treatment may be considered. Surgical evacuation of a compressive haematoma may be considered.

Malignant Middle Cerebral Artery Infarction (Fig. 2.34)

Definition and Clinical Features

Total middle cerebral artery infarction causing complete deficit and early disorders of consciousness (first 24–48 h) due to vasogenic oedema, causing elevation of intracranial pressure and ultimately death by uncal herniation.

Malignant infarction represents less than 1 % of all cerebral infarctions and is usually due to distal occlusion of an internal carotid artery or occlusion of the origin of the middle cerebral artery with poor collateral circulation. It occurs more frequently in young subjects with 80 % mortality in the absence of surgical treatment.

Imaging

Predictive elements of malignant progression of middle cerebral artery infarction: disorders of consciousness with complete deficit and total volume of abnormalities on diffusion-weighted sequence within the first 24 h $\geq$ 145 cc.

Treatment

Large hemicraniectomy plus opening of dura mater (Fig. 2.35).

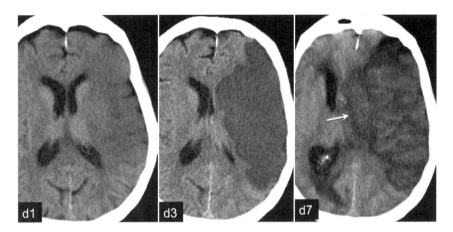

Fig. 2.34 CT scan of total left middle cerebral artery infarction on the 1st, 3rd and 7th days. Cerebral oedema has increased considerably over time with uncal herniation (*arrow*) and intracranial hypertension leading to the patient's death (malignant middle cerebral artery infarction)

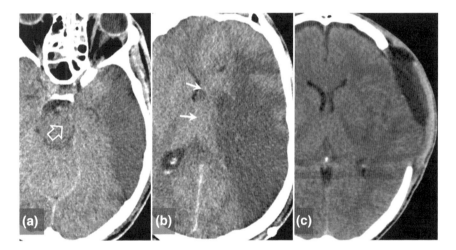

Fig. 2.35 CT of left malignant middle cerebral artery infarction causing uncal herniation (**a** *hollow arrow*) and midline shift (**b** *arrows*). Resolution of signs of herniation after decompression craniotomy (**c**)

Decompression craniotomy: reduction of the mortality rate from 80 to 20 % and reduction of sequelae.

Decompression craniotomy, as large as possible, must be performed urgently within the first 48 h (ideally 24 h) for malignant middle cerebral artery infarction in a patient under the age of 55, with an NIHSS score ≥ 16 (Ia subscore ≥ 1).

Subacute Outcome of Cerebral Infarction

Cortical Laminar Necrosis (Fig. 2.36)

Definition

Neuronal ischaemia due to hypoxia of the deep layers of the cortex associated with glial reaction and laminar deposits of lipid-laden macrophages. No haemorrhage.
    Aetiologies: all causes of cerebral hypoxia.

Imaging

• MRI

Cortical gyriform hyperintensity on T1 images and iso- or hyperintensity on T2 and FLAIR images. Gadolinium enhancement. No haemorrhagic hypointensity on T2-weighted GE sequences. Appearing 10–15 days after an ischaemic stroke. Partial resolution around the 3rd month. Persistence up until the 11th month.

Long-Term Outcome of Cerebral Infarction

Gliosis and Cystic Changes (Fig. 2.37)

Definition

Replacement of necrotic brain tissue by fluid (liquefaction necrosis) and/or glial fibres produced by astrocytes (astrocytic gliosis or glial scar due to neuroglial

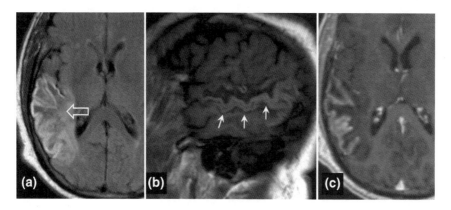

Fig. 2.36 MRI of a patient with history of right superficial middle cerebral artery infarction (**a** FLAIR sequence, *hollow arrow*). Cortical laminar necrosis with gyriform hyperintensity on T1-weighted images of postcentral gyrus and superior temporal gyrus associated with lipid deposits (**b** sagittal T1, *arrows*). Gyriform gadolinium enhancement (**c** gadolinium-enhanced axial T1-weighted sequence) due to disruption of the BBB

Fig. 2.37 Axial MRI FLAIR
sequence in a patient with a
history of left superficial
middle cerebral artery
infarction. Cortical atrophy
due to hypointense cystic
changes (*arrow*) and
hyperintense gliosis (*hollow
arrow*)

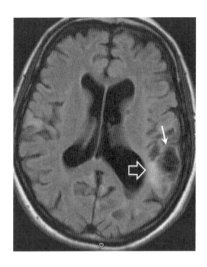

proliferation). The healing mode of necrotic tissue (gliosis or cystic changes)
varies from one subject to another and cannot be predicted at the initial phase.

Imaging

- Cystic changes: strong hyperintense signal on T2-weighted SE sequence and
  very hypointense (CSF signal) with more or less extensive hyperintense
  peripheral margin on FLAIR images.
- Cortical atrophy: enlargement of cortical sulci and basal cisterns. Frequently
  associated with leukoaraiosis. May or may not be associated with subcortical

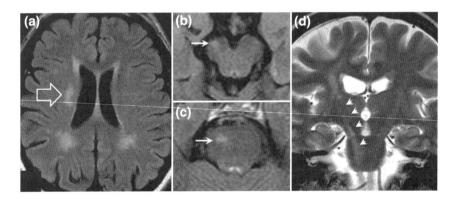

Fig. 2.38 MRI of Wallerian degeneration in a patient with a history of deep right middle
cerebral artery infarction (**a** *hollow arrow*, ischaemic scar with hyperintense signal on FLAIR
sequence). Degeneration of pyramidal tract giving a hyperintense signal on FLAIR sequence
(**b** and **c** axial section, *single arrow*) and T2-weighted SE imaging (**d** coronal section, *small
arrows*)

atrophy causing enlargement of the ventricular system and periventricular leukoaraiosis.
- Gliosis: hyperintense areas of cerebral parenchyma on T2-weighted SE images and FLAIR images, usually associated with some degree of cortical atrophy.

Wallerian Degeneration (Fig. 2.38)

Definition

Anterograde degeneration of axons and their myelin sheaths from destroyed neuronal cell bodies caused by multiple aetiologies: ischaemia, haemorrhage, tumour, demyelinating disorders, encephalitis.

Wallerian degeneration occurs away from the infarcted zone, along the course of nerve fibres derived from the ischaemic region, essentially involving large tracts, such as the pyramidal tract. It can also occur along all association fibres.

Imaging

Anomalies are visible on classical morphological imaging, four weeks after ischaemia. Atrophy is visible only after several months or several years.

- CT

Hypodensity ± atrophy of pyramidal tract in the brainstem.
Associated cortical and/or subcortical hypodense ischaemic scar in the middle cerebral artery territory.

- MRI

Hyperintense signal on T2-weighted SE images and FLAIR sequences along the pyramidal tract in the internal capsule (posterior limb), cerebral peduncle and brainstem. A coronal T2-weighted SE sequence is useful to follow signal anomalies along the tract. Possible cortical atrophy away from the zone of ischaemia.

Anomalies with decreased fractional anisotropy may be visible on diffusion-weighted images by the first week.

Aetiological Work-Up

First-Line Investigations

- Laboratory tests

  - At the acute phase of infarction: Complete blood count, platelets (haematological disease), PT, APTT, fibrinogen (prolonged APTT suggestive of circulating

anticoagulant, DIC, etc.), serum electrolytes, blood glucose, troponin.
In the presence of fever: CRP, blood cultures.

- Search for cardiovascular risk factors: fasting blood glucose and HbA1c, total cholesterol, LDL, HDL cholesterol and triglycerides.

- ECG: search for atrial flutter or fibrillation, signs of cardiac ischaemia, conduction disorders, ventricular hypertrophy.
- Carotid Doppler and transcranial Doppler looking for extracranial and intra-cranial stenoses, or signs of arterial dissection. Assessment of haemodynamic repercussions distal to the stenosis.
- Transthoracic echocardiography (TTE): determination of the size of heart chambers, study of global and segmental left ventricular function, search for valvular heart disease, ventricular thrombus or cardiac mass.

TTE can be combined with a contrast test to detect a right-left shunt related to patent foramen ovale.

TTE is not as accurate as transoesophageal echocardiography (TOE) for the diagnosis of cardiac emboli.

Second-Line Investigations

- TOE: search for segmental contractility disorder in favour of ischaemia, val-vular heart disease, vegetation suggestive of endocarditis, aortic arch plaques, intracardiac thrombus or spontaneous contrast, patent foramen ovale, atrial septal aneurysm.
- 24- or 48-hour Holter ECG monitoring: first-line examination when ECG monitoring was not performed at the acute phase, in patients with a history of palpitations and when imaging is highly suspicious of a cardioembolic origin.

The R-test allows ECG monitoring for 7 days. Only arrhythmias are recorded. The patient can trigger recording in the presence of palpitations.

Implantable Holter (Reveal®) is still under evaluation.

Special Cases

Young subjects: investigations for cerebral vasculitis and thrombophilia.

When imaging is suggestive of fibromuscular dysplasia associated with HT: search for associated renal artery stenosis.

Selected References

1. European Registers of Stroke Investigators (2009) Incidence of stroke in Europe at the beginning of the 21st century. Stroke 40:1557–1563
2. Bejot Y et al (2008) Trends in incidence, risk factors, and survival in symptomatic Lacunar stroke in Dijon, France, from 1989 to 2006: a population-based study. Stroke 39:1945–1951
3. Bejot Y et al (2007) Epidemiology of strokes. Impact on the treatment decision. Presse Med 36:117–127
4. Hiraga A (2009) Prediction of hemorrhagic transformation in ischemic stroke. Neuroepidemiology 33:266–267
5. Terruso V et al (2009) Frequency and determinants for hemorrhagic transformation of cerebral infarction. Neuroepidemiology 33:261–265
6. Paciaroni M et al (2008) Early hemorrhagic transformation of brain infarction: rate, prédictive factors, and influence on clinical outcome: results of a prospective multicenter study. Stroke 39:2249–2256
7. Vahedi K et al (2007) DECIMAL Investigators. Sequential-design, multicenter, randomized, controlled trial of early decompressive craniectomy in malignant middle cerebral artery infarction (DECIMAL Trial). Stroke 38:2506–2517
8. Vahedi K et al (2007) DECIMAL, DESTINY, and HAMLET investigators. Early decompressive surgery in malignant infarction of the middle cerebral artery: a pooled analysis of three randomised controlled trials. Lancet Neurol 6:215–222
9. Hofmeijer J et al (2009) HAMLET investigators. Surgical decompression for space-occupying cérébral infarction (the Hemicraniectomy After Middle Cerebral Artery infarction with Life-threatening Edema Trial [HAMLET]): a multicentre, open, randomised trial. Lancet Neurol 8:326–333
10. Takahashi S et al (1993) Hypoxic brain damage: cortical laminar necrosis and delayed changes in white matter at sequential MR imaging. Radiology 189:449–456
11. Sawada H et al (1990) MRI demonstration of cortical laminar necrosis and delayed white matter injury in anoxic encephalopathy. Neuroradiology 32:319–321
12. Mazumdar A et al (2003) Diffusion-weighted imaging of acute corticospinal tract injury preceding Wallerian degeneration in the maturing human brain. AJNR Am J Neuroradiol 24:1057–1066
13. Thomalla G et al (2005) Time course of wallerian degeneration after ischaemic stroke revealed by diffusion tensor imaging. J Neurol Neurosurg Psychiatry 76:266–268

Chapter 3
Territory Infarction

Territory infarction are the most common forms of cerebral infarction.

Contrary to lacunar infarcts, they are very rarely asymptomatic.

Clinical symptoms depend on the vascular territory affected.

The main aetiologies in subjects over the age of 50 are essentially arterial atherosclerosis or emboligenic heart disease. In younger subjects, the two main aetiologies are cardiac embolisms and arterial dissections. There are many other causes, all of which are very rare and, in almost 30 % of cases, no cause is found.

Atherosclerosis of Large and Medium-Sized Arteries

- 20 % of cerebral infarctions.
- Atherosclerosis most commonly affecting extracranial vessels (large arteries [Fig 3.1]: internal carotid artery, vertebral artery and basilar artery) and in 20–25 % of cases, the intracranial vessels (medium-sized arteries [Fig 3.2]: anterior, middle and posterior cerebral arteries and anterior choroidal artery).
- Mechanism of infarction: most commonly thromboembolic (thrombosis [role of platelets] secondary to stenosis and/or artery-to-artery atherosclerotic embolism) or more rarely haemodynamic.

Pathology

Damage of large elastic arteries and muscular arteries (internal carotid arteries, basilar artery, subclavian arteries) by lipid and fibrin deposits, often calcified and possibly leading to ulceration, intraplaque haemorrhage or thrombosis. A classification of atherosclerotic lesions has been proposed by Stary (Table 3.1).

Note that isolated atherosclerotic intracranial stenoses are rare in Caucasians and mainly occur in Black or Asian subjects.

G. Saliou et al., *Practical Guide to Neurovascular Emergencies*,
DOI: 10.1007/978-2-8178-0481-1_3, © Springer-Verlag France 2014

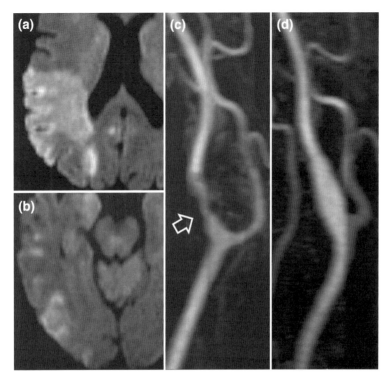

Fig. 3.1 Right superficial middle cerebral artery infarction: hyperintense signal on diffusion-weighted imaging (**a** and **b**) with embolic material from irregular stenosis of the right carotid artery (**c**, cerebral MR angiography: *hollow arrow*). Surgically revascularized stenosis (**d**)

Clinical Features

- Often elderly subject with one or several cardiovascular risk factors.
- Clinical signs depend on the arterial territory affected.
- MCA/ACA junctional infarction is sometimes observed in internal carotid artery occlusion.

Imaging

CT Angiography and MR Angiography

Proximal artery stenosis (carotid bifurcation, origin of vertebral arteries). Intra-cranial stenosis (especially the basilar artery, 1st segment of Circle of Willis arteries). Unlike post-radiation stenoses (Fig 3.3), atherosclerotic carotid artery

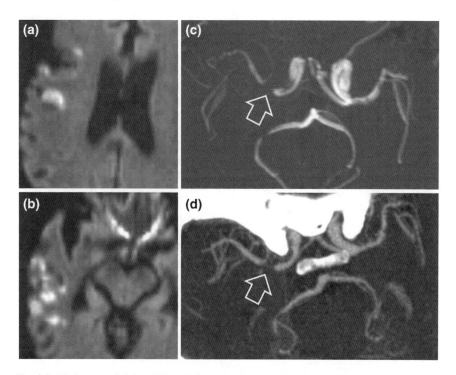

Fig. 3.2 Right superficial middle cerebral artery infarction (**a** and **b** diffusion-weighted sequences) in a subject with an intracranial atherosclerotic stenosis. Note the subocclusive stenosis of the origin of the right middle cerebral artery visualized by MRI (**c** TOF sequence, *hollow arrow*) and MR angiography (**d** *hollow arrow*)

Table 3.1 Classification of atherosclerotic lesions according to Stary

Lesion type	Term	Description
I	Isolated macrophage foam cells	Isolated macrophage foam cells within intima. No extracellular lipids.
II	Fatty streak	Layers of macrophage foam cells. Lipid-laden smooth muscle cells. Scattered extracellular lipid particles.
III	Pre-atheroma	Like type II with multiple extracellular lipid deposits forming small aggregates.
IV	Atheroma	Like type II with multiple massive confluent extracellular lipid deposits (lipid core).
V	Fibroatheroma	Like type IV with massive collagen deposits (fibrous cap) covering lipid core (type Va) with calcifications (type Vb).
VI	Complicated	Like type V with disruption of fibrous cap (VIa), intraplaque haemorrhage (VIb) or thrombosis (VIc).
VII	Fibrotic plaque	Massive intimal thickening with collagen (sclerosis); No or negligible amount of intracellular and extracellular lipids.

stenoses do not extend upstream into the common carotid arteries. Calcification of
the arterial wall at the level of the stenosis is often visible on CT scan.

Quantification of Carotid Artery Stenoses

Two methods are generally used:

- NASCET-ACAS method (NASCET: *North American Symptomatic Carotid
  Endarterectomy Trial*; ACAS: *Asymptomatic Carotid Atherosclerosis Study*):
  minimum diameter of the stenosis divided by the diameter of the healthy cervical internal carotid artery (Fig 3.4).
- ECST *(European Carotid Surgery Trial)* method: minimum diameter of the
  stenosis divided by the maximum diameter of the carotid bulb (Fig 3.5).

There is a correlation between the values estimated by the two methods
(Table 3.2). For tight stenoses, the values obtained by the two methods are very
similar.

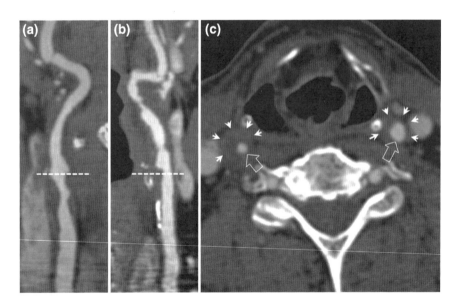

Fig. 3.3 Carotid CT angiography in a subject with a history of laryngeal cancer treated by
radiotherapy. Unlike atherosclerotic stenosis, post-radiation carotid artery stenosis involves the
distal third of the common carotid arteries and the origin of the internal carotid arteries in the
irradiated field (**a** and **b** CT angiography: common carotid artery below the dotted line, internal
carotid arteries above). Post-radiation thickening of the arterial wall is clearly visible on axial
sections (**c** axial section through the larynx and common carotid arteries at the level of maximum
stenosis), small lumen (*hollow arrows*) with significant thickening of carotid artery walls (*small
arrows*).

Fig. 3.4 NASCET-ACAS
method for stenosis
calculation: calculation with
reference to the healthy
cervical internal carotid
artery. %
stenosis = (C−A)/C × 100

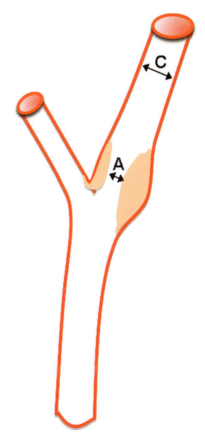

Treatment of Cerebral Infarction

- Emergency treatment:

  - Intravenous thrombolysis (sometimes intra-arterial) when indicated and in the absence of contraindications.
  - Aspirin (in the absence of associated haemorrhage) when thrombolysis is not possible or after thrombolysis.
  - Blood pressure control: maximum systolic blood pressure: 220 mmHg/maximum diastolic blood pressure: 110 mmHg, but no sudden lowering of blood pressure.
  - Prevention of venous thromboembolic events by low-molecular-weight heparin (high prophylactic dose) in patients with a motor deficit of a lower limb or unable to walk.

- Secondary prevention:

  - Correction of cardiovascular risk factors.
  - Antiplatelet therapy.

Fig. 3.5 ECST method for
stenosis calculation:
calculation with reference to
the largest diameter of the
carotid bulb. %
stenosis $= (B-A)/B \times 100$

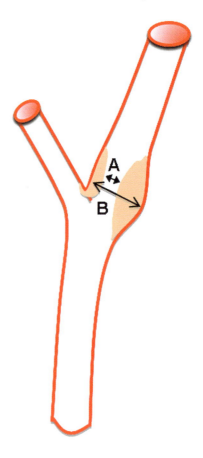

Table 3.2 Correlation between the percentage stenosis of arterial diameter according to the method used

NASCET–ACAS method (%)	30	40	50	60	70	80	90
ECST method (%)	65	70	75	80	85	91	97

NASCET North American symptomatic carotid endarterectomy trial
ACAS Asymptomatic carotid atherosclerosis study
ECST European carotid surgery trial

Treatment of Atherosclerotic Stenosis

In France, the standard treatment in addition to medical treatment, is surgery.

Indications for surgical carotid endarterectomy (degree of stenosis according to NASCET method)

Symptomatic carotid artery stenosis

• Major cause of stroke: risk $= 14$ %/year if stenosis >70 % (NASCET).

Surgery is very effective: risk = 4 %/year after endarterectomy (10 % absolute risk reduction).

- Surgical indications:
  - Atherosclerotic stenosis between 70 % and 99 %: surgery indicated.
  - For patients with a history of TIA or moderately large or resolving stroke: carotid artery surgery performed as soon as possible (<2 weeks) is more effective than delayed treatment.

Carotid artery Stenosis >70 % + Carotid TIA = EMERGENCY

- between 50 % and 69 %: surgery is indicated but with decreased benefit, particularly for women.
- carotid artery surgery not beneficial for stenoses less than 50 % and harmful and contraindicated for stenoses less than 30 %.

Asymptomatic carotid artery stenosis

Accounts for a low proportion of infarcts (2 %/year), but constitutes a marker of global vascular risk (risk of myocardial infarction > risk of cerebral infarction).

- No surgical indication when stenosis <60 %.
- For stenoses ≥60 %, studies comparing surgery and medical treatment only indicate similar results, but in favour of surgical treatment: 1 % absolute risk reduction.

The benefits of surgical treatment for asymptomatic stenoses ≥60 % are observed in the long term, after more than one year. The benefit has been much less clearly established for women.

Carotid angioplasty and stenting (still under evaluation)

This procedure can be proposed essentially when the surgeon considers surgery to be contraindicated for technical or anatomical reasons (contralateral recurrent laryngeal nerve paralysis, neck immobility, radiotherapy, tracheotomy, severe tissue lesions or inaccessible carotid artery stenoses).

Cardioembolic Infarction (Fig. 3.6)

Cardiac emboli: haemorrhagic transformation in up to 50 % of cases
Frequent aetiology: approximately 20 % of cerebral infarctions.

The aetiological diagnosis may sometimes be difficult as atherosclerosis is often associated: positive diagnosis when a potential cardiac source of embolism is demonstrated or exclusion of another cause of cerebral infarction.

About 20 % of patients with cardiac sources of embolism present another cause of infarction (especially elderly subjects).

Aetiologies

Atrial fibrillation (AF) (50 % of cases): mixed thrombus from the dilated left atrium or auricle (coagulating role). Less common: supraventricular arrhythmia, left atrial dilatation, heart failure, dilated cardiomyopathy, left ventricular wall motion abnormalities, endocarditis, right-left shunt (patent foramen ovale with or without atrial septal aneurysm: PFO–ASA, frequent anomaly, but its aetiological role remains controversial).

Clinical Features

Increased incidence with age. Clinical signs according to the arterial territory(ies) affected.

Frequently severe infarction, as often very extensive. High early and late mortality.

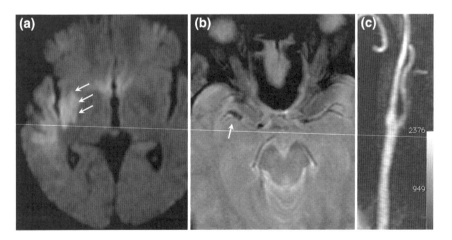

Fig. 3.6 Cardioembolic right middle cerebral artery infarction. Hyperintensity on diffusion-weighted imaging in the territory of the right MCA (**a** *triple arrow*). Note the hypointense blood clot in the MCA on the T2*-weighted sequence (**b** *arrow*). No visible stenosis in the right carotid bulb (**c**). Echocardiography revealed thrombus in the left atrium due to atrial fibrillation

Brain Imaging

Often more extensive and more often haemorrhagic infarction compared to other aetiologies.

MRI

Sometimes multiple lesions affecting several vascular territories in the case of multiple micro-emboli.

Thrombus visible as endoluminal hypointensity on T2*-weighted sequences.

Hypointensity on T2-weighted GE sequences in the presence of associated haemorrhage must be systematically investigated.

MR Angiography

In theory, no visible stenosis in extracranial and intracranial arteries, but in practice, these patients often present associated atherosclerosis (age of patients with AF = age of patients with atherosclerosis). Intracranial vascular occlusion sometimes visible.

Cardiac Imaging

Doppler echocardiography (transthoracic or transoesophageal) (Fig 3.7)

- Atrial dilatation (AF risk factor), decreased LVEF, presence of intracardiac thrombus, post-ischaemic wall motion abnormalities (risk factor for thrombus formation).
- Visualization of atrial septal aneurysm with left to right Doppler flow or passage of microscopic gas bubbles from the right atrium to the left atrium on bubble test while performing Valsalva manoeuvre.

Outcome

Early: sometimes very early (by the 6th hour) and frequent haemorrhagic transformation (up to 50 % of cardioembolic infarcts followed by CT scan).

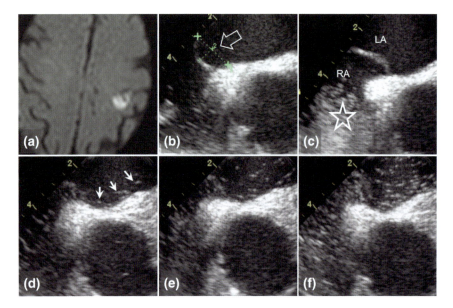

Fig. 3.7 Cardioembolic infarction due to paradoxical embolism in a female subject with PFO-ASA. The atrial septal aneurysm is clearly visible on echocardiography (**b** *hollow arrow*) bulging into the right or left atrium with heart beat (**b** and **c**). During the bubble test, no passage of bubbles from right atrium to left atrium (**c** RA right atrium, LA left atrium), bubbles are clearly visible as hyperechogenic spots in the right atrium (**c** *star*). During the Valsalva manoeuvre, passage of bubbles from right atrium to left atrium (**d** *arrows*) with progressive filling of left atrium (**e** and **f**), accounting for the mechanism of paradoxical embolism during exercise. Reprinted with kind permission from Dr. Christophe Bressolle

Treatment

- Emergency thrombolysis or thrombectomy when indicated in the acute phase.
- Anticoagulant or antiplatelet treatment may be considered (efficacy of heparin has not been demonstrated):
  - effective anticoagulation initially by heparin (unfractionated or LMWH) in the absence of disorders of consciousness, if small infarct, no significant haemorrhage on imaging and high risk of early recurrent embolism, followed by oral anticoagulants.
  - in all other cases, aspirin 300 mg/day is indicated for 10 days to 1 month, followed by oral anticoagulation (after resolution of the bleeding risk) with a target INR between 2 and 3.
- Blood pressure control: maximum systolic blood pressure: 220 mmHg/maximum diastolic blood pressure: 110 mmHg.
- Correction of cardiovascular risk factors.

- Prevention of venous thromboembolic events by LMWH (high prophylactic dose) in patients with a motor deficit of a lower limb or unable to walk (and treated by aspirin).
- Cardiological treatment when necessary.

Dissection of Extracranial Carotid and Vertebral Arteries

90 % of dissections (Fig 3.8).
Dissection of one neck artery may mask dissection of another artery: 20 % of multiple dissections (Fig 3.9)!

Pathophysiology

- Subintimal or subadventitial tear of the arterial wall causing mural haematoma. Increased artery diameter with decreased lumen diameter.
- Usual site of dissection:

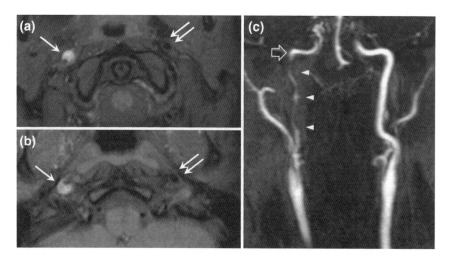

Fig. 3.8 Dissection of the right cervical internal carotid artery in a young woman. Note the mural haematoma which is hyperintense on fat saturation T1-weighted images (**a** and **b** single *arrows*) and enlargement of the dissected artery compared to the contralateral internal carotid artery (**a** and **b** *double arrows*). MR angiography shows the dissection as irregular, flame-like carotid artery stenosis (**c** *arrowheads*). The dissection typically stops at the site of entry of the carotid artery in the carotid canal (**c** *hollow arrow*).

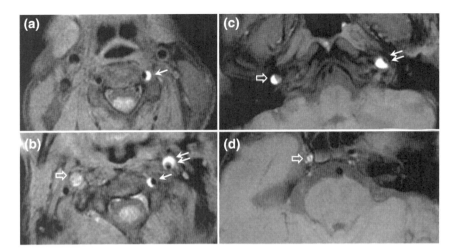

Fig. 3.9 Young subject injured in a road accident two weeks earlier. Persistent neck pain and a TIA. Note the multiple dissections of the cervical part of the internal carotid arteries (**b** and **c**) extending into the petrous (**c**) and cavernous parts (**d**) and the associated left vertebral artery dissection (**a** and **b** *single arrow*). Dissection with mural haematoma (fat saturation T1-weighted sequence: hyperintense crescent) in left vertebral artery (*single arrow*), left internal carotid artery (*double arrows*) and right internal carotid artery (*hollow arrow*). Carotid artery dissections remain extradural as they do not extend beyond the origin of the ophthalmic artery in the cavernous sinus

- cervical part of internal carotid artery (most common): 1 or 2 cm after the origin of the internal carotid artery.
- vertebral: V3 > V2 > V1 segments (possibly related to the marked mobility of the cervical spine at V3 segment).

Clinical Features

Two percent of all cerebral infarctions (20–25 % in subjects under the age of 45). Mean age: 40–45 years. Look for risk factors (traumatic, see above).

- Local clinical signs: may be isolated or precede the transient ischaemic attack or stroke. Neck pain, headache or facial pain (90 %) ipsilateral to the dissection. In the case of carotid artery dissection, painful Horner's syndrome in approximately 50 % of cases (ptosis, miosis, enophthalmos), ipsilateral to the dissection, due to compression of cervical sympathetic fibres, is highly suggestive of the diagnosis.

  Unilateral pulsatile tinnitus (10 %), hypoglossal nerve palsy (5 %).

- Downstream consequences (cerebral or ocular): transient ischaemic attacks or stroke in 60 % of cases. Haemodynamic or thromboembolic ischaemia. Infarction generally occurs during the week following onset of local signs, but sometimes after a longer period, up to 1 month. Transient monocular blindness is much less common (mainly of haemodynamic origin).
- Sometimes asymptomatic.
- Low risk of relapse (approximately 1 % per year), rarely at the same site as the initial dissection.

Aetiology

Traumatic (rare) following an unusual effort, sudden flexion and extension neck movements or, much more frequently, spontaneous: acute phenomenon probably enhanced by a more fragile arterial wall due to fibromuscular dysplasia, connective tissue disease (<5 % of dissections: Ehlers-Danlos syndrome, Marfan syndrome, osteogenesis imperfecta, pseudoxanthoma elasticum), upper respiratory tract infections (during the previous month). There is a continuum between traumatic and spontaneous aetiologies; the patient often reports a history of more or less minor trauma.

Imaging

Note: when an extracranial artery is dissected, always check for the absence of intracranial extension and associated dissection of another artery.

Cerebral infarction in the territory of the dissected artery (60 % of cases).

Possibility of watershed strokes due to haemodynamic stenosis related to mural haematoma.

CT

Crescent-shaped enlargement and hyperdensity (mural haematoma) of a carotid artery compared to the contralateral side; the diameter of the carotid arteries is physiologically almost always the same on both sides (constitutional asymmetry of carotid arteries is very rare and always associated with a smaller carotid canal in the skull base).

Increased diameter is more difficult to confirm for vertebral arteries, as these arteries may be physiologically asymmetrical (the left vertebral artery is often dominant). Cerebral infarction may occur in the territory of the dissected artery.

MRI

Axial sequences perpendicular to carotid arteries and axial or coronal sequences for vertebral arteries. Mural haematoma is hyperintense on T1-weighted images (by the 3rd day) or proton density images, ideally with fat saturation (Fat Sat T1 sequence). Possible contrast enhancement of the thickened dissected wall. Infarction in the territory of the dissected artery. During the first three days of the acute phase, mural haematoma is sometimes difficult to identify, as it is isointense on T1-weighted images.

MR Angiography or CT Angiography

Long, irregular and extensive (characteristic) stenosis. Sometimes "candle flame" occlusion (suggestive but not specific, as it may be due to terminal internal carotid artery occlusion with retrograde thrombus).

A double lumen appearance is rare, but pathognomonic. Arterial dilatation or blister-like or fusiform aneurysm may be observed.

Outcome

Clinical: favourable, without sequelae in 70–90 % of cases and a mortality rate of 2–5 %. Less than 1 % of patients relapse at 1 year. Favourable long-term prognosis at 10 years: 85 % survival, 75 % of patients are independent. Relapsing ischaemic attacks despite antiplatelet therapy in 5 % of patients: search for residual dissection, haemodynamic stenosis, a new dissection or underlying fibromuscular dysplasia.

Imaging: 60 % complete revascularization, 20 % occlusion. 90 % stabilization at three months. Residual aneurysms in 10 % cases (good prognosis).

Treatment

No randomized study has been performed.

Strict bed rest in the case of distal haemodynamic consequences beyond the dissection (transcranial Doppler flow in MCA).

Pure Extracranial Dissection: Antithrombotic Treatment

Two treatment options can be proposed and should take into account the state of the artery, the presence or absence of ischaemic signs, the time since onset of symptoms:

– effective anticoagulation by heparin (target APTT between 2 and 3 times control values), in the absence of disorders of consciousness, small infarction and in the absence of haemorrhagic transformation. Oral anticoagulant therapy for 3–6 months, followed by antiplatelet therapy, depending on the results of MR angiography.
– aspirin 300 mg/day.

At the acute phase, intravenous thrombolysis is possible for extracranial dissection with infarction. Intra-arterial thrombectomy and/or thrombolysis can sometimes be indicated.

In the Case of Intracranial Extension of the Dissection

(more frequent for vertebral artery dissection): sometimes no antithrombotic treatment. Anticoagulation is possible but only after formally excluding meningeal haemorrhage by MRI and LP (aspirin is often preferred). Total treatment duration according to course of arterial healing.

Regular Doppler ultrasound follow-up.

Intracranial Dissection (Figs. 3.10 and 3.11)

Pathophysiology

Often subadventitial dissection of an intracranial artery. The arterial tear can result in meningeal haemorrhage (10–20 % of cases) or, more rarely, intraparenchymal haematoma and also arterial pseudoaneurysm. The mural haematoma can be responsible for infarction by occlusion or stenosis of the dissected vessel. Internal carotid artery dissection is intracranial when it extends beyond the origin of the ophthalmic artery. The extracranial—intracranial limit for vertebral arteries is more difficult to define due to the marked variability of the origin of the division branches, particularly the PICA.

Clinical Features

Thunderclap headache in the case of meningeal haemorrhage. TIA or sudden neurological deficit in the case of stroke or cerebral haemorrhage.

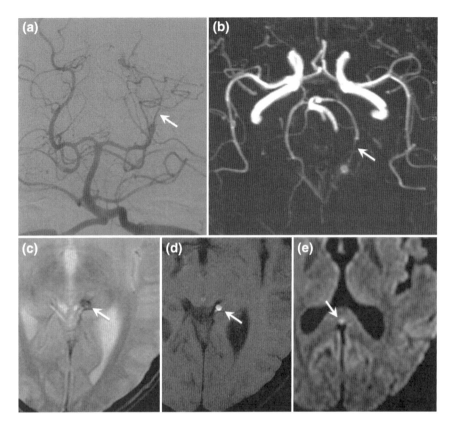

Fig. 3.10 Intracranial dissection of the 2nd segment of the left posterior cerebral artery. Arteriography (**a** *arrow*, frontal view of vertebrobasilar system) and intracranial MR angiography (**b** *arrow*, inferior view) demonstrating irregular stenosis of the dissected artery. The mural haematoma is hypointense on MRI T2-weighted GE sequences (**c** *arrow*), hyperintense on T1-weighted sequences (**d** *arrow*). On diffusion-weighted images, minimal ischaemic zone of the splenium of the corpus callosum (**e** *arrow*)

Aetiology

Spontaneous. Predominantly located on the supraclinoid internal carotid artery or vertebrobasilar system: termination of the vertebral artery from the origin of the posterior inferior cerebellar artery extending to the basilar artery and junction of the 1st and 2nd segments of the posterior cerebral artery due to trauma to the free edge of the tentorium cerebelli.

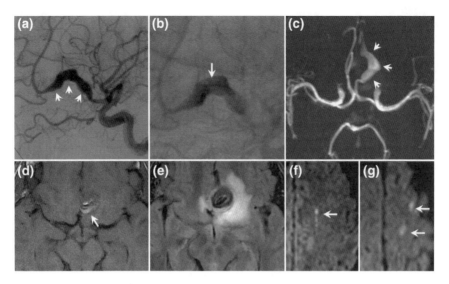

Fig. 3.11 Intracranial dissection of the 2nd segment of the left anterior cerebral artery. Left carotid arteriography (**a** *triple arrows*, lateral view of left ACA and internal carotid artery) and intracranial MR angiography (**c** *triple arrows*, *top view*) demonstrating a fusiform aneurysm of the dissected artery. Typical double lumen appearance observed on the arteriogram with a double concentric movement in the fusiform aneurysm (**b** *arrow*). The mural haematoma is hypointense on MRI on T1-weighted sequences (**d** *arrow*). Presence of peripheral oedema, hyperintense on FLAIR imaging due to mass effect of the mural haematoma on the adjacent cerebral parenchyma (**e**). On diffusion-weighted images, minimal ischaemic zone in the left frontal watershed zone (**f** and **g** *arrows*)

Imaging

Difficult diagnosis.

CT

Hypodensity in the ischaemic territory. Hyperdense appearance of the cortical sulci due to meningeal haemorrhage. Intraparenchymal hyperdensity in the presence of haematoma. Hyperdensity and enlargement of the dissected artery related to mural haematoma. Stenosis/arterial occlusion or fusiform dilation and/or pseudoaneurysm on contrast-enhanced CT.

MRI

Enlargement and hyperintense signal on T1-weighted images (gradient-echo and spin-echo) and hypointense on T2-weighted GE sequences (gradient-echo) of the dissected artery related to mural haematoma (pathognomonic). Restriction of territorial diffusion in the presence of associated infarction. On MR angiography (TOF or after gadolinium injection), occlusion or irregular stenosis, fusiform dilation and/or pseudoaneurysm of the dissected segment.

Arteriography

Rare visualization of a double lumen (pathognomonic) or more frequently irregular stenosis and/or fusiform dilatation of the dissected artery. Identification of a pseudoaneurysm situated outside of an arterial bifurcation with pooling of contrast agent in the aneurysm.

Treatment

Absence of consensus. Absolute contraindication to aspirin or anticoagulants during the acute phase in the presence of meningeal haemorrhage. After having **formally excluded meningeal haemorrhage by MRI and LP**, aspirin and even anticoagulant therapy for a total duration of 3–6 months. Severe risk of intracranial haemorrhage in patients treated with antiplatelet or anticoagulant therapy.

In the case of meningeal haemorrhage and/or pseudoaneurysm, consider emergency endovascular exclusion of the dissected segment (high risk of severe spontaneous haemorrhage). Some authors propose conservative management with the use of a stent or coils for basilar artery dissection (no consensus), but high risk of secondary thrombosis. Surgical ligation of vertebral artery can sometimes be proposed.

Selected References

1. Stary HC et al (1995) A definition of advanced types of atherosclerotic lesions and a histological classification of atherosclerosis: a report from the committee on vascular lesions of the council on arteriosclerosis American heart association. Circulation 92:1355–1374
2. Brott TG, Halperin JL et al (2011) ASA/ACCF/AHA/AANN/AANS/ACR/ASNR/CNS/SAIP/ SCAI/SIR/SNIS/SVM/SVS guideline on the management of patients with extracranial carotid and vertebral artery disease: executive summary: a report of the American College of Cardiology Foundation/American Heart Association Task Force on Practice Guidelines, and the American Stroke Association, American Association of Neuroscience Nurses, American Association of Neurological Surgeons, American College of Radiology, American Society of Neuroradiology, Congress of Neurological Surgeons, Society of Atherosclerosis Imaging and Prevention, Society for Cardiovascular Angiography and Interventions, Society of Interventional Radiology, Society of NeuroInterventional Surgery, Society for Vascular Medicine, and Society for Vascular Surgery. Developed in collaboration with the American Academy of

Neurology and Society of Cardiovascular Computed Tomography. Catheter Cardiovasc Interv. 2013 Jan 1 81(1):E76—123

3. Bousser MG, Mas JL (2009) Traité de neurologie. Accident vasculaire cérébraux. Edition Dion 91:423–441

4. Bousser MG, Mas JL (2009) Traité de neurologie. Accident vasculaire cérébraux. Edition Dion 387:515–531

5. Bousser MG, Mas JL (2009) Traité de neurologie. Accident vasculaire cérébraux. Edition Dion 91:443–469

6. Kocaeli H et al (2009) Spontaneous intradural vertebral artery dissection: a single-center experience and review of the literature. Skull Base 19:209–218

7. Kim BM et al (2008) Management and clinical outcome of acute basilar artery dissection. AJNR 29:1937–1941

8. Ahn JY et al (2006) Endovascular treatment of intracranial vertebral artery dissections with stent placement or stent-assisted coiling. AJNR 27:1514–1520

Chapter 4
Watershed Infarction

Watershed infarction is due to ischaemia in the border zones of two adjacent arterial territories or between the deep and superficial territories of the middle cerebral artery (Fig. 4.1).

Aetiology

Low cardiac output (resuscitation after cardiocirculatory arrest or shock regardless of the cause, severe heart failure) or severe extracranial (Fig. 4.2) or intracranial arterial stenosis (Fig. 4.3) or atherosclerotic occlusion or dissection.

A low output state can cause bilateral multifocal lesions (especially in the carotid/vertebrobasilar watershed territory), while arterial occlusion causes elongated subcortical ischaemic lesions in the watershed territory of two adjacent arteries. The most common form of watershed infarction consists of frontoparietal lesions between the anterior cerebral artery territory and the middle cerebral artery territory.

Diagnosis

Radiological: ischaemia in the watershed zone of two adjacent arteries.

Clinical Features

Watershed infarctions are often associated with haemodynamic disorders (severe hypotension, cardio circulatory failure causing bilateral infarction; hypotension, bradycardia with tight stenosis or occlusion of an internal carotid artery causing unilateral infarction).

G. Saliou et al., *Practical Guide to Neurovascular Emergencies*,
DOI: 10.1007/978-2-8178-0481-1_4, © Springer-Verlag France 2014

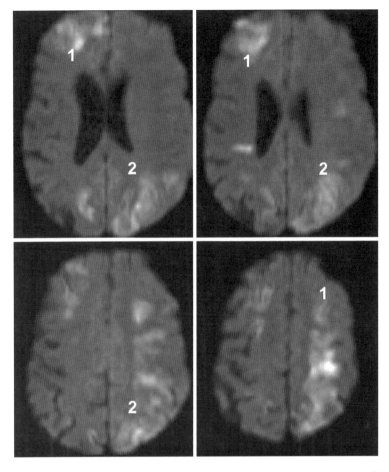

Fig. 4.1 Patient who experienced cardiac arrest responsible for low output state. Cerebral ischaemia involving all border zones of the brain (*1* border zone between anterior and middle cerebral arteries, *2* border zone between middle and posterior cerebral arteries)

Initial transient symptoms preceding the onset of a completed deficit, trans-cortical aphasia and early seizures are overrepresented in such infarctions.

Subjects are usually elderly, with generalized vascular disease. The patient may experience an initial loss of consciousness, anterior TIAs due to haemodynamic phenomena (standing, hypotension), progressive or fluctuating onset of symptoms, limb-shaking syndrome contralateral to the stenosis, frequent seizures.

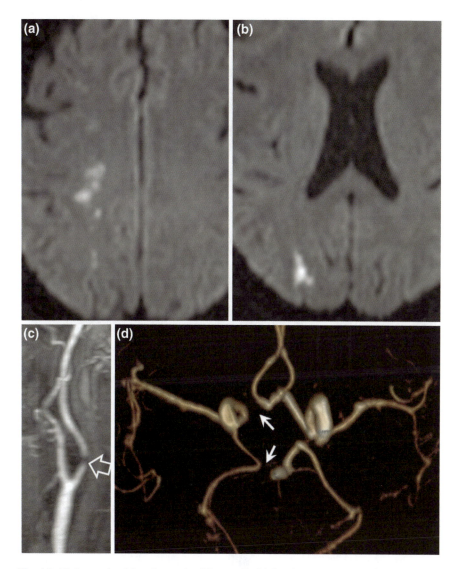

Fig. 4.2 Right anterior (**a**) and posterior (**b**) watershed infarction (**a**) secondary to sub-occlusive carotid artery stenosis (**c** *hollow arrow*). Brain TOF MR angiography (**d**) reveals a normal variant with hypoplasia of the first segment of the right anterior and posterior cerebral arteries (**d** *arrows*) accounting for absence of collateral flow to the right internal carotid artery via the Circle of Willis

Superficial Watershed Infarction

Watershed infarction occurs at anastomoses of terminal branches of two superficial territories (watershed stroke).

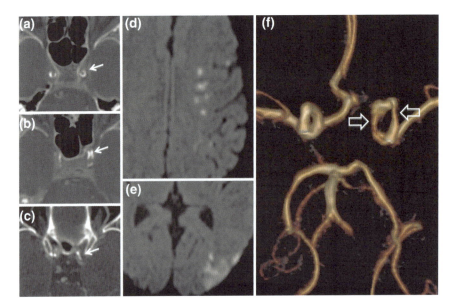

Fig. 4.3 Left watershed infarction secondary to intracranial atherosclerotic stenosis. Brain CT angiography (**a**, **b**, **c**) demonstrates internal carotid artery calcifications predominantly on the left (*single arrows*) causing serial stenoses. MRI diffusion-weighted images (**d** and **e**) show hyperintensities related to cerebral ischaemia in the anterior (**d**) and posterior (**e**) watershed territories. Intracranial MR angiography (**f** TOF sequence, bottom view) visualizes major stenoses of the cavernous left internal carotid artery (*hollow arrows*)

Anterior Watershed Infarct (between superficial ACA and MCA territories) (Fig. 4.4)

Clinical features similar to those of ACA infarction: infarction predominantly involving the subcortical white matter causes predominantly proximal weakness of the controlateral lower limb and motor aphasia when the lesion is left-sided. Infarction confined to the cortex causes proximal brachial hemiparesis. In this case, bilateral lesions can cause bibrachial paresis (man-in-the-barrel syndrome).

Posterior Watershed Infarct (between superficial internal carotid artery territory and superficial PCA territory) (Fig. 4.5)

Predominantly brachiofacial hemihypesthesia, hemiparesis with the same distribution, homonymous hemianopsia, fluent aphasia (left-sided lesion), anosognosia and spatial hemineglect (right-sided lesion). Often bilateral after cardiac arrest or profound hypotension.

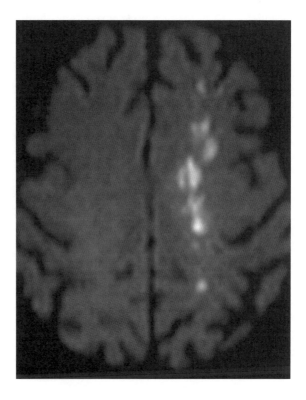

Fig. 4.4 Anterior watershed infarct. Hyperintensity on diffusion-weighted images in the border zone of the superficial territories of the anterior cerebral artery and the middle cerebral artery

Subcortical Watershed Infarction

Subcortical watershed infarction occurs in the border zone between a superficial territory (pial branches) and a deep territory (penetrating branches), in the absence of collateral circulation (border-zone infarction), especially watershed infarction between superficial and deep territories of the MCA.

Clinical features: predominantly brachiofacial hemiparesis, hemihypesthesia with the same distribution, homonymous hemianopsia, neuropsychiatric disorders.

Limb Shaking Syndrome

Transient ischaemic attack due to low cardiac output associated with tight stenosis or occlusion of the contralateral internal carotid artery, characterized by brief stereotyped repetitive involuntary movements of a limb while standing, with no electroencephalographic abnormalities. It requires emergency management in a neurovascular unit to prevent infarction (especially watershed infarction) and emergency carotid artery surgery in the presence of stenosis.

Fig. 4.5 Posterior watershed infarct. Hyperintensity on diffusion-weighted images in the border zone of the superficial territories of the internal carotid artery (ACA and MCA) and posterior cerebral artery

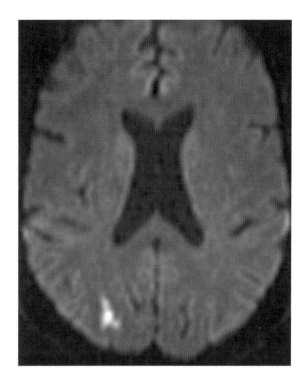

Imaging

CT

Cortical and subcortical hypodensity in a watershed territory. Intracranial or extracranial arterial stenosis detected on CT angiography with frequent arterial calcifications.

MRI

Cortical and subcortical hyperintensity on FLAIR and diffusion-weighted images with decreased ADC in the watershed territory. On perfusion-weighted imaging, increased MTT and TTP, decreased CBV and CBF, often more extensive than the hyperintense territory on FLAIR imaging (penumbra).

Cerebral MR Angiography

Tight stenosis or occlusion usually of an internal carotid artery in the case of an arterial cause. On fat saturation T1-weighted images, hyperintensity in the arterial wall if dissection with eccentric lumen (except in the case of occlusive dissection).

TREATMENT

- Strict bed rest.
- Platelet antiaggregants: aspirin.
- In the case of small infarction or repeated TIAs related to subocclusive stenosis, consider effective anticoagulation with heparin (target APTT between 1.5 and 2.5 times control values).
- Maintenance sufficient blood pressure (approximately 140/90 mmHg). Surgical treatment of internal carotid artery stenosis if indicated.

Selected Reference

1. Joinlambert C et al (2012) Cortical border-zone infarcts: clinical features, causes and outcome. J Neurol Neurosurg Psychiatry 83(8):771–775

Chapter 5
Transient Ischaemic Attacks

Definition

A transient ischaemic attack (TIA) is defined as 'a brief episode of neurological dysfunction due to focal cerebral or retinal ischaemia with symptoms typically lasting less than one hour and without evidence of acute infarction' according to the ANAES 2004 guidelines.

TIA is a medical emergency and requires immediate management to avoid cerebral infarction. The same applies to any focal deficit, regardless of its duration, which has resolved at the time of examination.

Clinical Features

- Symptoms suggestive of carotid TIA:

  - Monocular blindness (of haemodynamic or embolic origin)
  - Speech disorder (aphasia)
  - Unilateral motor and/or sensory deficit involving the face and/or limbs, often predominantly brachiofacial; these symptoms usually indicate ischaemia in the carotid territory but, in the absence of other signs, it is impossible to determine whether the attack is of carotid or vertebrobasilar origin.

- Symptoms suggestive of vertebrobasilar TIA:

  - Bilateral or alternating sensory and/or motor deficit, involving the face or limbs
  - Loss of vision in the homonymous visual hemi-field (homonymous hemianopsia) or in both homonymous visual hemi-fields (cortical blindness); homonymous hemianopsia can also occur in carotid TIAs.
  - Associated suggestive symptoms: vertigo, diplopia, dysarthria, swallowing disorders, loss of balance.

G. Saliou et al., *Practical Guide to Neurovascular Emergencies*,
DOI: 10.1007/978-2-8178-0481-1_5, © Springer-Verlag France 2014

Imaging

Brain imaging may be normal. Focal or limited hyperintensity is often visible on diffusion-weighted images: the frequency of abnormalities increases with the duration (>1 h) and the type of symptoms (aphasia and motor deficit) and decreases with the time lag before MRI (abnormalities resolve within 7–15 days). Old territory or lacunar infarcts may be visualized on FLAIR sequences.

The aim of brain and cardiac imaging is to identify the aetiology of the TIA: extracranial or intracranial vascular stenosis (Fig. 5.1), mechanical heart valve thrombosis, endocarditis or aortic dissection.

Differential Diagnosis

- Migraine aura (positive phenomena [scintillating scotoma, phosphene], aura progression, symptoms followed by headache).
- Partial epileptic seizure (positive signs, myoclonus).
- Hypoglycaemia.
- Other neurological diagnoses: brain tumour, transient global amnesia, cerebral haemorrhage, etc.
- Other non-neurological diagnoses: vertigo of ENT origin, syncope, psychosomatic disorder, etc.

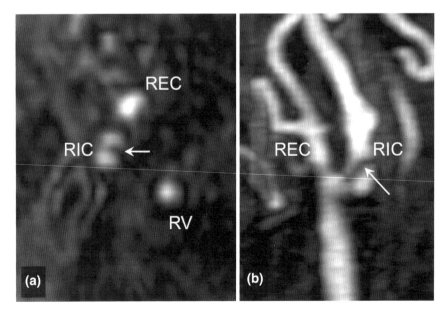

Fig. 5.1 Patient with right carotid TIA. MR angiography (**a** axial section, **b** sagittal reconstruction) shows unstable plaque of right carotid bulb with endoluminal fragment (*arrow*). *REC* right external carotid artery, *RIC* right internal carotid artery, *RV* right vertebral artery

Identification of Patients at Risk of Complications

About 10 % of patients with TIA subsequently experience stroke over the next 3 months, and half of them within 48 h.

TIA patients have a global vascular risk, i.e. a risk of stroke, myocardial infarction and/or vascular death of about 6 % per year.

Clinical Criteria

ABCD2 score

- A for *Age*. If > 60 years = 1 point.
- B for *Blood pressure*. If systolic blood pressure > 140 mmHg or diastolic blood pressure > 90 mmHg = 1 point.
- C for *Clinical deficit*. If unilateral motor deficit = 2 points, speech deficit without motor deficit = 1 point.
- D for *Duration*. If symptoms last > 60 min = 2 points, 10 to 59 min = 1 point, < 10 min = 1 point.
- D for Diabetes: 1 point.
- Overall sum gives the total score:
- **For a score between 0 and 3**: low risk estimated at 3 % at 3 months. ECG, MRI or CT should be performed promptly.
- **For a score between 4 and 5**: moderate risk estimated at 10 % at 3 months. The patient should be admitted for investigation.
- **For a score between 6 and 7**: high risk estimated at 8 % at 48 h. Emergency admission of the patient to a neurovascular intensive care unit.

However, a low score cannot exclude onset of a stroke: a young person with transient monocular blindness and headache caused by carotid dissection has a 0 score! Regardless of the score, TIA remains a diagnostic and therapeutic emergency (secondary prevention).

Aetiology of TIA

Stroke risk within 3 months following a TIA is highest when the TIA is due to atherosclerotic stenosis (20 % at 3 months); a cardio embolic cause is associated with an intermediate risk (11.5 %).

Radiological Criteria

Following a TIA, the presence of ischaemic lesions on brain CT or MRI diffusion-weighted sequence is an independent predictive factor for stroke in the short term.

Selected References

1. Albucher JF et al (2005) Clinical practice guidelines: diagnosis and immediate management of transient ischemic attacks in adults. Cerebrovasc Dis 20:220–5
2. Purroy F et al (2007) Patterns and predictors of early risk of recurrence after transient ischemic attack with respect to etiologic subtypes. Stroke 38:3225–9
3. Donnan GA et al (2006) Patients with transient ischemic attack or minor stroke should be admitted to hospital: for. Stroke 37:1137–8
4. Bousser MG, Mas JL (2009) Traité de neurologie Accidents vasculaires cérébraux. Ed Doin 71:1147–1153

Chapter 6
Lacunar Infarcts and Small-Vessel Disease

Lacunar infarcts represent 25 % of all cerebral infarctions.

Lacunar cavity due to ischaemia, less than 15 mm in largest diameter, usually due to occlusion of a single penetrating artery of the brain with a diameter less than 400 μm.

Aetiology

Essentially chronic disease of the walls of small arteries and arterioles. Lipohyalinosis of penetrating arteries, secondary to hypertension, diabetes, age and all chronic small-vessel diseases. Lacunar infarcts occur in the subcortex, basal ganglia, periventricular white matter, centrum semiovale and brainstem (pons). Leukoaraiosis is frequently associated. Lacunar infarcts may sometimes be due to cardiac or atheromatous embolism.

Clinical Features

Most lacunar infarcts are silent.

Lacunar infarcts can have a sudden onset but in 30 % of cases, the onset is progressive, fluctuating or stepwise and preceded by a TIA.

Classical lacunar syndromes:

- Pure motor hemiparesis: pure motor deficit involving all three body areas; lacunar infarct in the internal capsule or pons.
- Ataxic hemiparesis: motor deficit with cerebellar ataxia affecting one side of the body; lacunar infarct in the posterior limb of the internal capsule or brainstem.
- Pure sensory syndrome: subjective and/or objective sensory deficit affecting one side of the body, involving the three body areas; thalamic lacunar infarct.
- Dysarthria/clumsy hand: facial and tongue paralysis, clumsy hand but no weakness; pontine lacunar infarct.

G. Saliou et al., *Practical Guide to Neurovascular Emergencies*,
DOI: 10.1007/978-2-8178-0481-1_6, © Springer-Verlag France 2014

- Mixed sensorimotor syndrome: same symptoms as pure sensory syndrome with ipsilateral pyramidal dysfunction or paralysis; lateral thalamic lacunar infarct involving the internal capsule.

Good functional prognosis and low risk of early relapse (0–4 % in the 1st month) but long-term risk of relapse similar to that of other types of infarction with a risk of cognitive disorders: 15 % risk of dementia after 9 years of follow-up.
More than one half of relapses are non-lacunar!

Aetiological Work-Up

Laboratory tests:
Complete blood count, platelets, PT, APTT, fibrinogen, electrolytes, glucose, 24 h proteinuria.
Systematic ECG.
Systematic carotid Doppler and transcranial Doppler.
TTE: looking for LVH suggestive of longstanding HBP and segmental abnormalities of ventricular contraction that can predispose to cardiac microemboli.
Funduscopy to diagnose and assess the impact of HBP.

Imaging (Fig. 6.1)

CT

CT can be normal. Deep focal hypodensities in the white matter or basal ganglia indicating old lacunar infarcts.
Diffuse periventricular hypodensities when associated with leukoaraiosis.

MRI

- Variable signal depending on the age of the lesion; gradual progression towards a "hole" in the brain parenchyma:

  - acute lesion: focal hyperintensity on FLAIR and T2 images and normal or decreased ADC. Perfusion-weighted imaging often shows minor and very focal changes with increased MTT and decreased CBV; no penumbra.
  - subacute lesion: focal hyperintensity on FLAIR and T2 images and increased ADC.

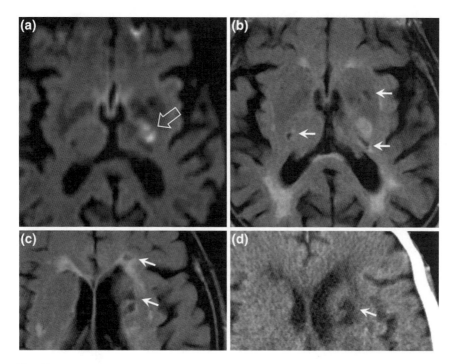

Fig. 6.1 Hyperintense lacunar infarct in the left lateral sulcus on diffusion-weighted images (**a** *hollow arrow*). It is associated with multiple lacunar infarct sequelae as "holes" in the brain parenchyma, hypointense on FLAIR imaging with a more or less intense hyperintense corona (**b** and **c** *arrows*) and hypodense on CT (**d** *arrow*)

- chronic lesion: T2 hyperintensity and FLAIR hypointensity ± hyperintense crown; T1 hypointensity.
- Diffuse periventricular FLAIR hyperintensities when associated with leukoaraiosis.
- Frequently associated with micro-haemorrhages visualized as T2* hypointensities <10 mm (haemorrhagic lacunae).

Treatment

No specific study. Treatment identical to that of atherothrombotic ischaemic strokes:

- Intravenous thrombolysis, if indicated (the small size of a lacunar infarct is not considered to be a contraindication).
- Aspirin.
- Blood pressure control +++

- Correction of other cardiovascular risk factors.
- Prevention of venous thromboembolic events in patients with motor deficit of a lower limb or unable to walk.

Chapter 7
Rare Cerebral Angiopathies

Cerebral angiopathies are responsible for cerebral infarction and/or cerebral haemorrhage.

Cerebral Vasculitis (Fig. 7.1)

Definition

- Inflammatory lesion of the vessel wall due to various causes: infectious, systemic, primary, toxic. Vascular necrosis may be observed. Frequency: systemic > infectious/toxic > primary.
- Involvement of large, medium-sized or small vessels depending on the aetiology.
- The definitive diagnosis is based on histological examination of brain biopsy, which is rarely performed. The diagnosis is therefore generally based on a body of evidence: clinical, laboratory (high CSF cell count) and radiological. Diagnosis is difficult, particularly when cerebral vasculitis reveals systemic vasculitis or when vasculitis is confined to the central nervous system.

Clinical Features

The most common, although nonspecific symptom is acute or rapidly progressive headache (rarely thunderclap type). Focal neurological deficit, seizures, impairment of consciousness.

G. Saliou et al., *Practical Guide to Neurovascular Emergencies*,
DOI: 10.1007/978-2-8178-0481-1_7, © Springer-Verlag France 2014

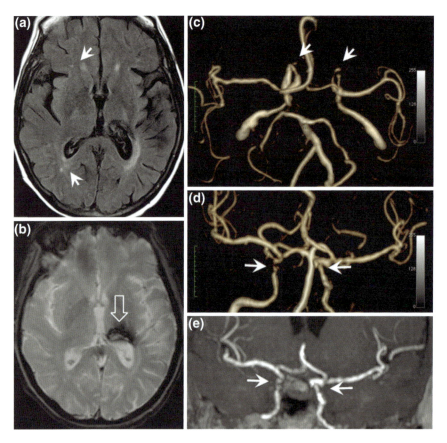

Fig. 7.1 Cerebral vasculitis in a 50-year-old female with a history of TIA. MRI FLAIR sequence (**a** *arrows*): focal white matter hyperintensities. Left thalamic hypointensity on T2* sequence (**b** *hollow arrow*) related to old haematoma. Intracranial TOF MR angiography (**c**, **d** and **e**): multiple irregularities and arterial stenoses mainly involving terminal internal carotid arteries (**c**, **d** and **e** *arrows*)

Aetiologies

- Infectious: purulent meningitis, tuberculosis (Fig. 7.2), VZV, HSV, HIV, syphilis (tertiary), mycotic and parasitic.
- Systemic: Takayasu arteritis, polyarteritis nodosa (PAN), giant cell arteritis, Wegener's granulomatosis, connective tissue diseases (systemic lupus erythematosus (Fig. 7.3), scleroderma), Behçet's disease, Sjögren's syndrome, rheumatoid arthritis.
- Toxins: opioids, heroin, cocaine, crack.

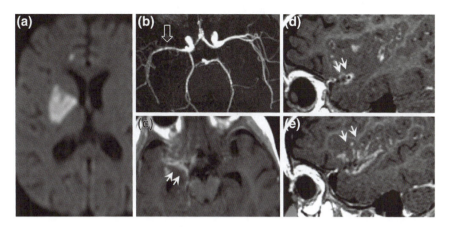

Fig. 7.2 Tuberculous cerebral vasculitis in a child with right deep middle cerebral artery infarction (**a** diffusion sequence). Stenoses and irregularities of right middle cerebral artery on the TOF sequence (**b** *hollow arrow*) with perivascular and meningeal contrast enhancement (**c**, **d** and **e** *double arrows*) related to infection

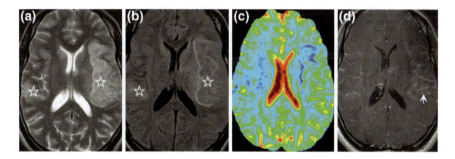

Fig. 7.3 Systemic lupus erythematosus in a 26-year-old patient. Recent bilateral middle cerebral artery cerebral infarction (**a** [T2] and **b** [FLAIR]: *stars*). Decreased ADC in ischaemic territories (**c** decreased ADC is shown in *blue*). Diffuse pial contrast enhancement after gadolinium injection (**d** *arrow*)

- Isolated primary vasculitis of CNS (Fig. 7.4): isolated CNS vasculitis is rare, characterized by a nonspecific lymphocytic or necrotic granulomatous inflammatory infiltrate (also called cerebral granulomatous angiitis). It is diagnosed after exclusion of other causes of cerebral vasculitis.

Note: In SLE, the cerebral ischaemic lesion is more often caused by emboligenic lupus cardiomyopathy than by cerebral vasculitis.

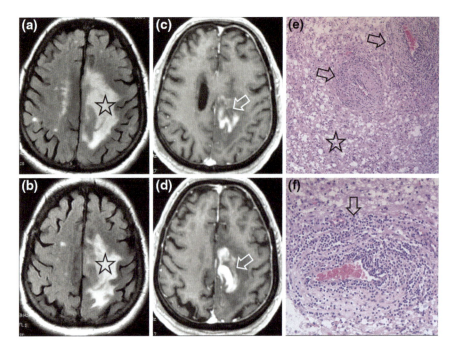

Fig. 7.4 Recent progressive right hemiplegia in a 74-year-old female patient. MRI shows oedematous lesions on FLAIR sequence (**a** and **b** *stars*) with cortical contrast enhancement (**c** and **d** *hollow arrows*). Histological diagnosis of primary central nervous system vasculitis: thickening of arterial walls (**e** and **f** *arrows*) and intravascular and perivascular T lymphocyte infiltrate with necrosis of adjacent cerebral parenchyma (**e** *star*). *By courtesy of Dr. M. Levasseur, hôpital d'Orsay*

Aetiological Work-Up

Laboratory tests:

- routine: CBC, platelets, serum protein electrophoresis, CRP;
- immunological: ANA, anti-DNA, ANCA, circulating anticoagulant, anti-phospholipid antibodies, rheumatoid factor, cryoglobulin, complement, angio-tensin-converting enzyme;
- serology: herpes virus, varicella-zoster, hepatitis viruses, HIV, Lyme disease;
- lumbar puncture.

Funduscopy or even fluorescein angiography.

ENT examination: look for evidence of Wegener's granulomatosis.

Brain biopsy: only biopsy can provide the definitive diagnosis in primary CNS vasculitis and should be performed whenever aggressive treatment is considered.

Imaging

CT

Multiple intraparenchymal hypodensities corresponding to ischaemic sequelae. Intraparenchymal or cortical sulcus hyperdensity in the presence of cerebral or meningeal haemorrhage.

MRI

Multiple stenoses of intracranial and extracranial arteries on TOF sequences and cerebral MR angiography. Multiple focal, mostly subcortical hyperintensities on T2 and FLAIR images corresponding to ischaemic sequelae. Isolated or multiple focal hyperintensities on diffusion-weighted images with decreased ADC related to recent ischaemia. Possible contrast enhancement and thickening of vessel walls related to mural inflammation, especially visible on thin sections (2 or 3 mm) and with fat saturation (Fig. 7.5). Leptomeningeal contrast enhancement (more clearly visible on T1 SE sequences and less clearly visible on gradient-echo sequences such as 3D MPR sequences) and hyperintensity of cortical sulci on FLAIR sequences related to inflammation of leptomeningeal vessels. Signs of focal pachymeningitis may sometimes be observed.

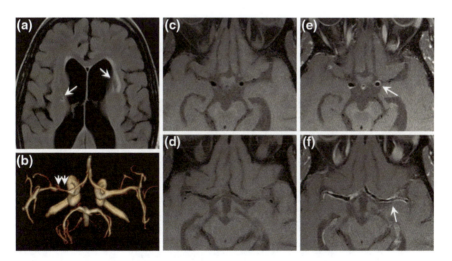

Fig. 7.5 Cerebral vasculitis in a 56-year-old female patient. MRI FLAIR sequence (**a** *arrow*) visualizes focal hyperintensities corresponding to old deep infarcts. On TOF sequence (**b** posterosuperior view, *double arrows*), severe stenosis of M1 segment of right middle cerebral artery. Diffuse contrast enhancement of arterial wall, clearly visible on T1 sequences on thin sections with fat saturation, before (**c** and **d**) and after gadolinium injection (**e** and **f** *arrow*)

Arteriography

Succession of segmental stenoses and/or arterial irregularities ± associated with interposed fusiform dilatations. Vascular occlusions.

Parenchymographic defect in hypoperfused or ischaemic zones. May be associated with distal aneurysms.

Imaging

Consensus for at least long-term steroid therapy (oral and possibly with initial boluses), usually in combination with immunosuppressive therapy (monthly bolus or daily oral cyclophosphamide, azathioprine, methotrexate).

Duration of treatment according to therapeutic response (the main outcome measure must be defined at the start of treatment: clinical, imaging, CSF ?).

Generally associated with a poor prognosis.

Non-Inflammatory CNS Small-Vessel Disease

CADASIL (Fig. 7.6)

Definition and Clinical Features

CADASIL means "*Cerebral Autosomal Dominant Arteriopathy with Subcortical Infarcts and Leukoencephalopathy*". Autosomal dominant disorder of small

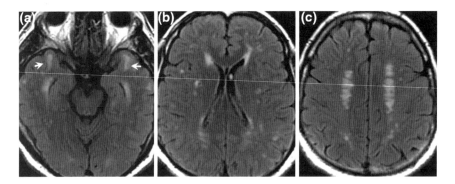

Fig. 7.6 CADASIL (Notch 3 mutation) in a 47-year-old patient. FLAIR sequence: diffuse hyperintensities of the periventricular and subcortical white matter. Constant involvement of anterior poles of the temporal lobes with white matter hyperintensities (**a** *arrow*) on FLAIR sequence

perforating arteries associated with migraine with aura (one-third of cases), recurrent subcortical infarcts, mood disorders (apathy, severe depression, episodes of melancholia and mania), pseudobulbar syndrome and dementia. Mutation in the Notch 3 gene. The vascular disease is responsible for white matter ischaemia. Death around the age of 60 years, about twenty years after the first ischaemic sign.

Investigations

In patients with a family history or personal history of migraine with aura, recurrent lacunar infarcts, severe leukoaraiosis on imaging: screening for Notch 3 gene mutations (more than 100 mutations have been identified).

Imaging

MRI

Diffuse nonspecific leukoencephalopathy with constant involvement of anterior poles of temporal lobes and subcortical ischaemia, visualized as hyperintensities on FLAIR and T2 images. Dilated Virchow-Robin spaces. Multiple lacunar infarcts. Diffuse microbleeds, seen as focal T2* hypointensities.

Treatment

No known treatment.
Usual stroke management.

Sneddon's Syndrome (Fig. 7.7)

- Multifocal infarcts and livedo racemosa in young subjects.
- Most frequent symptom: headache. May mimic migraine with aura.
- Investigations: screening for circulating anticoagulant, antiphospholipid, anti-cardiolipin, and anti-beta2GP1 antibodies.

Imaging

MRI: multiple focal white matter hyperintensities on T2-weighted sequences. Pseudo-multiple sclerosis appearance on MRI.

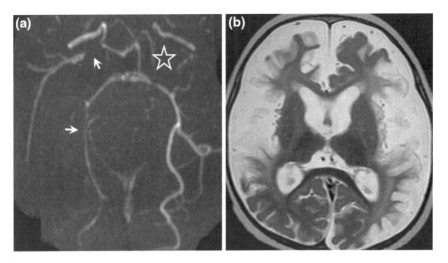

Fig. 7.7 Sneddon's syndrome with antiphospholipid antibodies in a young patient associated with cerebral vasculitis responsible for infarction and livedo racemosa. MRI shows extensive involvement with multiple proximal vascular stenoses of the carotid and vertebrobasilar systems (**a** TOF sequence, *inferior view, arrows*) with left middle cerebral artery occlusion (**a** *star*). On T2-weighted SE sequences, multiple sequelae of extensive infarcts with diffuse parenchymal atrophy

SUSAC'S Syndrome (Fig. 7.8)

Also called SICRET syndrome *(Small Infarction of Cochlear, Retinal and Ence-phalic Tissue)*. It is a microangiopathy responsible for the occlusion of small retinal, cerebral and cochlear vessels. More common in young women. Symptoms comprise small cerebral infarcts, impaired hearing and vision.

Investigations

Funduscopy and fluorescein angiography (small retinal infarcts), audiometry to detect cochlear lesions.

Imaging

MRI: multiple scattered small infarcts. Typical lesion of corpus callosum involving central fibres with relative sparing of peripheral fibres (in contrast with multiple sclerosis): multiple rounded "snowball" central callosal focal hyperintensities (while corpus callosum anomalies are peripheral in MS).

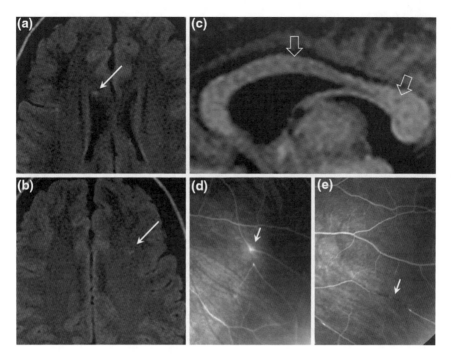

Fig. 7.8 34-year-old female with Susac's syndrome. MRI FLAIR sequence shows focal periventricular white matter hyperintensities (**a** and **b** *arrows*) with suggestive central callosal lesions (**c** *hollow arrows, central callosal holes* on T1). Fluorescein angiography demonstrates fluorescein leakage (**d** *arrow*) and lesions suggestive of peripheral vasculitis (**e** *arrow, vascular occlusion*). *Funduscopic views by courtesy of Dr. Yvan de Monchy, hôpital Bicêtre*

Syndromes Related to Col 4A1 Gene Mutations (Fig. 7.9)

Definition

Hereditary autosomal dominant lesions related to mutation of the Col 4A1 gene encoding procollagen type $4\alpha1$.

Several phenotypes have been described:

- hereditary infantile hemiparesis with leukoencephalopathy and retinal arteriolar tortuosity;
- leukoencephalopathy and recurrent cerebral haemorrhage;
- HANAC (Hereditary Angiopathy with Nephropathy, Aneurysms and muscle Cramps) syndrome: haematuria with bilateral renal cysts associated with systemic angiopathy, intracranial aneurysms and muscle cramps.

Life-threatening in the case of cerebral haemorrhage.

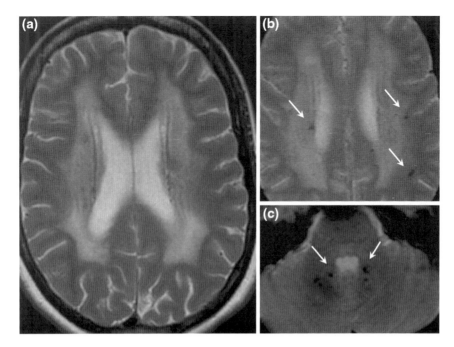

Fig. 7.9 45-year-old patient with vestibular neuronitis, pyramidal syndrome and mild attention deficit. Funduscopy showed arterial tortuosity. Family history of renal failure in both parents. Col 4a1 gene mutation was confirmed by molecular genetics. Appearance suggestive of very extensive, nonspecific white matter disease associated with microbleeds. *By courtesy of Dr. Elisabeth Auffray Calvier, hôpital de Nantes*

Imaging

MRI

Nonspecific cerebral small-vessel disease possibly associated with intracranial aneurysms of the terminal internal carotid arteries and haemorrhagic sequelae in the form of microbleeds. Intraparenchymal haematoma if recent haemorrhage. Possible dilatation of Virchow-Robin spaces.

Systemic Investigations

- Funduscopy: presence of arteriolar tortuosity.
- Laboratory tests: elevated creatine kinase. Possible renal failure.

Reversible Cerebral Vasoconstriction Syndrome (RCVS) (Fig. 7.10)

RCVS is not strictly speaking a form of small-vessel disease, but a vasomotor disorder.

Definition

Clinical and radiological syndrome combining headache with multiple segmental stenoses involving medium-sized and small vessels reversible in less than three months. Predominantly observed in females (two-thirds of cases).

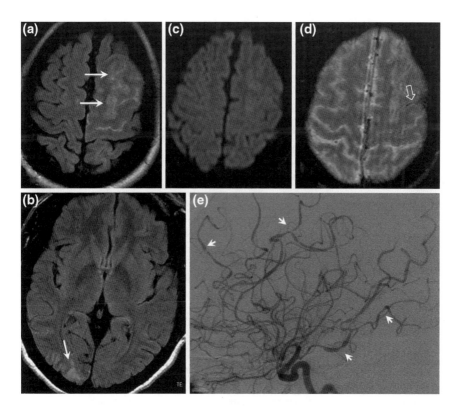

Fig. 7.10 Reversible cerebral vasoconstriction syndrome in a postpartum woman. Predominant cortical involvement with hyperintensities on FLAIR sequences (**a** and **b** *arrows*). Normal diffusion-weighted images (**c**). Minimal meningeal haemorrhage seen as a hypointensity in a left frontal cortical sulcus on T2-weighted GE images (**d** *hollow arrow*). Arteriography: combination of multiple segmental stenoses and dilatations giving a suggestive "string of sausages" appearance (**e** *small arrows*)

Aetiology: postpartum, toxaemia of pregnancy, toxins (cannabis = leading toxic cause [30 % of cases], cocaine, ecstasy, crack, amphetamine, LSD), medications (serotonin reuptake inhibitors, nasal decongestants, sympathomimetics, antimigraine drugs), catecholamine-secreting tumours (phaeochromocytoma) and idiopathic.

Clinical Features

Main symptom: recurrent thunderclap headache over several days in 94 % of patients, possibly. associated with meningeal (22 %) or intraparenchymal haemorrhage (6 %). More rarely, seizures, reversible posterior leukoencephalopathy, TIA or infarction (<5 % of cases).

Investigations

Laboratory tests: urine toxin screen (cannabis, cocaine, amphetamines).

In the presence of HT, assay of methoxylated derivatives in urine to detect possible phaeochromocytoma.

Lumbar puncture can contribute to the differential diagnosis with vasculitis.

Carotid Doppler and transcranial Doppler looking for dissection, sometimes associated with this syndrome, and a reversible increase of velocities suggesting arterial spasm.

Imaging

CT

Hyperdensity of cortical sulci (localized cortical meningeal haemorrhage) and/or intraparenchymal (haematoma).

CT Angiography

Nonspecific appearance of segmental stenoses of medium-sized and large vessels (vasculitis).

MRI

TOF sequence: multiple intracranial arterial stenoses, sometimes not visible on this sequence (3 Telsa MRI is more sensitive to detect these stenoses). Stenoses may be better seen on gadolinium-enhanced TOF sequences (improved visibility of distal small arteries). Focal meningeal haemorrhage visualized as hyperintensity in cortical sulci on FLAIR sequences and hypointensity on T2 gradient-echo sequences. Intraparenchymal haematoma. Focal parenchymal hyperintensity on diffusion-weighted images (low ADC) and FLAIR images in the presence of ischaemia. White matter hyperintensity on FLAIR sequences with normal ADC, predominantly in the occipital region when associated with posterior reversible leukoencephalopathy. Possible meningeal or intraparenchymal contrast enhancement (if disruption of blood–brain barrier).

Arteriography

Succession of regular segmental stenoses and arterial dilatations with "string of sausages" appearance. No venous anomaly. Arteriography must be repeated three months later: diagnosis is confirmed when anomalies have resolved and angiography is normal.

Treatment

No randomized study has been performed.

Elimination of the cause when due to a toxin. Intravenous nimodipine (Nimotop®) in the acute phase (1–2 mg/hour depending on blood pressure), followed by oral nimodipine (30–60 mg every 4 h depending on blood pressure). Analgesics if headache.

Prognosis is poorer in the presence of stroke (particularly haemorrhagic stroke).

Fabry's Disease (Fig. 7.11)

X-linked genetic lysosomal storage disease due to mutation of the GLA gene. More than 300 mutations have been described to date and 1 out of 15 are *de novo* mutations. This mutation is responsible for alpha-galactosidase A deficiency, resulting in accumulation of glycosphingolipids in lysosomes of many cell types.

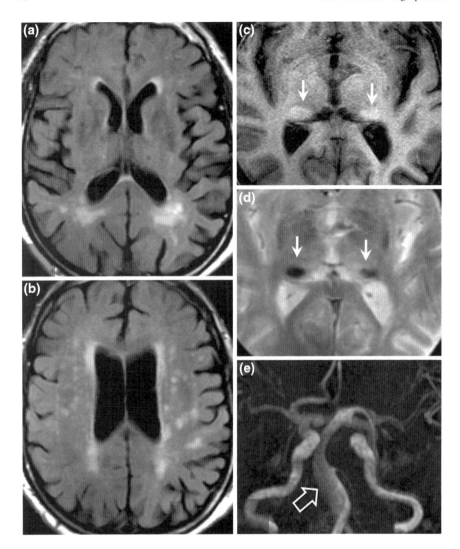

Fig. 7.11 67-year-old patient with Fabry's disease. Suggestive cerebral lesion with nonspecific cerebral small-vessel disease on FLAIR sequences (**a** and **b**), abnormally hyperintense signal on T1-weighted images and hypointense on T2* images of pulvinars due to microcalcifications and local hypoperfusion (**c** and **d** *arrows*) and dolichoectasia of the basilar artery (**e** TOF sequence of the Circle of Willis, *hollow arrow*). *By courtesy of Dr. M. Kocheida, hôpital Raymond-Poincaré, Garches*

Clinical Features

Estimated prevalence between 1/117,000 and 1/40,000. Mean age at diagnosis is 29 years with a diagnostic delay of about 14 years in men and 17 years in women.

Initial symptoms consist of paroxysmal acute attacks with paraesthesia and/or burning sensations in the extremities (normal electromyogram) triggered by fatigue, stress, rapid changes in temperature or relative humidity (tingling and/or burning sensations affecting the palms and soles) during childhood, possibly associated with fever or arthralgia or oedema.

Angiokeratomas, hypohydrosis with intolerance to extreme temperatures due to a hypothalamic lesion, abdominal pain, diarrhoea, fatigue, deafness and/or tinnitus, proteinuria, mitral valve prolapse may be observed.

Corneal lesions with cornea verticillata (whorl-like corneal deposits). Without treatment, severe complications appear around the 4th or 5th decade: end-stage kidney disease, cardiac arrhythmias and conduction disorders, hypertrophic cardiomyopathy and cardiac or cerebral ischaemic complications.

Infiltration of the brainstem, spinal cord, amygdalae and hypothalamus causing hypotensive episodes.

Less often, cerebral infarction due to progressive stenosis of small arteries due to deposits and intimal fibrosis and/or platelet hyperaggregability, accounting for about 5 % of cryptogenic ischaemic strokes in men before the age of 55. High stroke relapse rate: 76 % in hemizygous males and 86 % in heterozygous females.

Hypertensive cerebral haemorrhages may also be observed.

Laboratory Diagnosis

- In men: assay alpha-galactosidase A enzyme activity.
- In women (residual enzyme activity): genotyping.

Imaging

Six percent of patients with normal brain MRI report a history of TIA symptoms.

Relative nonspecific small-vessel leukoencephalopathy (76 % of patients), increasing with age, not correlated with clinical symptoms.

Late involvement of basal ganglia (47 % of patients).

Frequent dolichoectasia of basilar artery (glycosphingolipid deposits in smooth medial muscle cells) possibly responsible for the higher incidence of posterior strokes (60 % of patients versus 20 % in the general population).

Hyperintensity of pulvinars on T1-weighted sequences (microcalcifications and local hypoperfusion): specific but late sign.

Treatment

Severe natural history due to renal and cardiac complications.

Enzyme replacement therapy allows clearance of renal, cardiac and skin deposits and improvement of brain metabolism but with no proven efficacy on the course of leukoencephalopathy and stroke prevention.

Moyamoya (Figs. 7.12 and 7.13)

Definition

Japanese term meaning "puff of smoke" related to the initial arteriographic description: stenosis or even terminal internal carotid artery occlusion with dilatation of lenticulostriate arteries, with a cloudy appearance (nonspecific term, giving no absolute indication of the aetiology of the small-vessel disease).

Distal stenosis of internal carotid arteries and proximal segments of anterior and middle cerebral arteries leading to obstruction, with development of a collateral network. The vertebrobasilar circulation is rarely involved.

Peak incidence in 5-year-old children and 40-year-old adults. Sex ratio: two women for 1 man. Incidence in Europe: 1/1,000,000 (10 times more common in the Japanese population).

Clinical Features

- Related to cerebral ischaemia: stroke, TIA, seizures. Ischaemic symptoms may be precipitated by dehydration.
- Related to neoangiogenesis (late) and collateral circulation phenomena: haemorrhage (intracerebral, intraventricular and subarachnoid) due to the fragility of collateral vessels, pseudomigrainous headache due to the development of transdural collateral vessels (dilatation of meningeal and leptomeningeal collateral arteries).
- Suzuki's 6-stage classification:

  - grade I: narrowing of terminal internal carotid arteries;
  - grade II: initiation of collateral vessels;
  - grade III: intensification of collateral vessels (deep vessels, responsible for moyamoya appearance) and further stenosis of internal carotid arteries;
  - grade IV: development of collateral network from the external carotid artery;
  - grade V: intensification of collateral circulation from external carotid artery and regression of collateral vessels responsible for moyamoya appearance;
  - grade VI: terminal internal carotid artery occlusion and disappearance of collateral vessels responsible for moyamoya appearance.

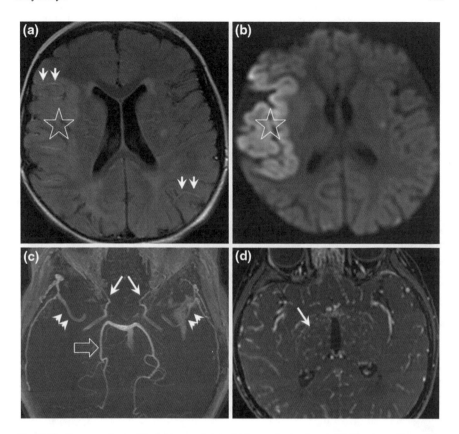

Fig. 7.12 Young patient with right superficial middle cerebral artery infarction (**a** and **b** *star*) in the setting of moyamoya disease. Abnormally clear visualization of the leptomeningeal network on FLAIR sequence (**a** *double arrows*) due to the well developed collateral circulation (ivy sign). Note stenosis of both internal carotid arteries (**c** *long arrows*) and absence of visualization of MCA and ACA on the TOF sequence. Abnormally clear visualization of middle meningeal arteries derived from the external carotid artery and contributing to the leptomeningeal blood supply to the brain (**c** *double arrows*) Posterior vertebrobasilar circulation is free of stenosis (**c** *hollow arrow*). After contrast injection, abnormally clear visualization of lenticulostriate arteries as punctate hyperintensities (**d** gadolinium-enhanced T1-weighted sequence, *arrow*) displaying the characteristic "puff of smoke"

Aetiologies

Moyamoya disease (primary, mainly in Asia): idiopathic (children), familial varieties are rare.

Moyamoya syndrome (secondary): atherosclerosis, post-radiation (radiotherapy for brain or head and neck tumour), sickle-cell disease, type I neurofibromatosis, Down syndrome (trisomy 21).

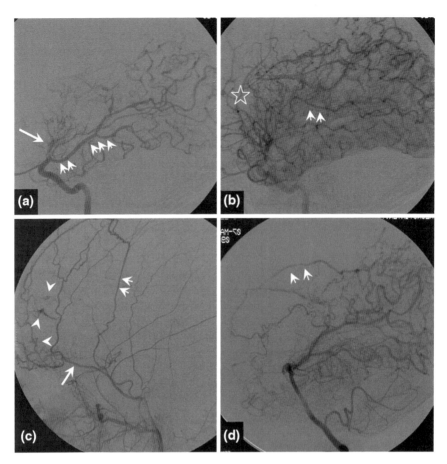

Fig. 7.13 Arteriography in a patient with grade V moyamoya according to Suzuki's classification (**a** and **b** lateral view of internal carotid artery at arterial and parenchymal phases, **c** lateral view of external carotid artery, **d** lateral view of vertebrobasilar system). Distal left internal carotid artery occlusion, terminating as anterior choroidal artery (**a** *arrow*) and posterior communicating artery (**a** *double arrows*) prolonged by the posterior cerebral artery (**a** *triple arrows*). The development of the leptomeningeal network provides collateral circulation to the middle cerebral artery (b: double arrows) and anterior cerebral artery (**b** *star*) territories. The external carotid artery supplies the brain via transosseous and transdural vessels (**c** *arrow heads*) derived from the superficial temporal artery (**c** *simple arrow*) and middle meningeal artery (**c** *double arrows*). The vertebrobasilar circulation is not affected, contributing to the leptomeningeal collateral circulation (**d** *double arrows*)

Investigations

Functional imaging such as positron emission tomography (PET): decreased regional blood flow and vascular reserve.

The stroke risk appears to be related to the decreased vascular reserve: PET results can be useful to determine the indication for surgical revascularization.

Imaging

CT

Focal or systematized hypodensities related to ischaemic sequelae.
Hyperdensity in the case of recent haemorrhage.

MRI

Areas of focal or territorial ischaemia. Hypointensity on T2-weighted gradient-echo sequences related to old or recent bleeding. On perfusion-weighted imaging: prolonged mean transit time (MTT) and time to peak (TTP) associated with the development of collateral vessels.

Cerebral blood volume (CBV) may be decreased in the case of poor collateral circulation or recent ischaemia or normal in the presence of a good collateral circulation. On TOF sequences, terminal internal carotid artery stenosis or even occlusion extending into the proximal segment of anterior and middle cerebral arteries. Possible wall contrast enhancement of the stenotic arteries. Very good visualization of distal branches of the external carotid artery (middle meningeal artery and superficial temporal artery). Enlargement of lenticulostriate arteries of the basal ganglia associated with the development of anterior choroidal collateral vessels, more clearly visible on gadolinium-enhanced 3D T1-weighted sequences. Linear cortical hyperintensities on FLAIR images associated with dilatations of the leptomeningeal collateral circulation and decreased cortical blood flow (ivy sign). Possible contrast enhancement of the leptomeningeal collateral circulation.

Treatment

Treatment of the cause in the case of secondary moyamoya. Surgical revascularization techniques depending on the lesions (burr holes, anastomosis between internal and external carotid arteries).

Selected References

1. Küker W (2007) Cerebral vasculitis: imaging signs revisited. Neuroradiology 49:471–479
2. Bousser MG, Biousse V (2004) Small vessel vasculopathies affecting the central nervous system. J Neuroophthalmol 24:56–61
3. Biousse V, Bousser MG (1998) Angiitis of the central nervous system in systemic diseases. Rev Med Interne 19:415–426
4. Bousser MG, Mas JL (2009) Traité de neurologie. Accident vasculaire cérébraux. Edition Dion 561–578
5. Chabriat H et al (2009) Lancet Neurol 8:643–653
6. Joutel A et al (1996) Notch3 mutations in CADASIL, a hereditary adult-onset condition causing stroke and dementia. Nature 383(6602):707–710
7. Chabriat H et al (1998) Patterns of MRI lesions in CADASIL. Neurology 51:452–457
8. Aladdin Y et al (2008) The Sneddon syndrome. Arch Neurol 65:834–835
9. Susac JO (2004) Susac's syndrome. AJNR Am J Neuroradiol 25(3):351–352
10. Susac JO, Murtagh FR, Egan RA, Berger JR, Bakshi R, Lincoff N, Gean AD, Galetta SL, Fox RJ, Costello FE, Lee AG, Clark J, Layzer RB, Daroff RB (2003) MRI findings in Susac's syndrome. Neurology 61(12):1783–1787
11. Plaisier E et al (2007) COL4A1 mutations and hereditary angiopathy, nephropathy, aneurysms, and muscle cramps. N Engl J Med 357:2687–2695
12. Gould DB et al (2006) Role of COL4A1 in small-vessel disease and hemorrhagic stroke. N Engl J Med 6(354):1489–1496
13. Vahedi K et al (2003) Hereditary infantile hemiparesis, retinal arteriolar tortuosity, and leukoencephalopathy. Neurology 14(60):57–63
14. Ducros A et al (2007) The clinical and radiological spectrum of reversible cerebral vasoconstriction syndrome. A prospective series of 67 patients. Brain 130:3091–3101
15. Clavelou P et al (2006) Manifestations neurologiques de la maladie de Fabry. Rev Neurol 162:569–580
16. Zarate YA, Hopkin RJ (2008) Fabry's disease. Lancet 18(372):1427–1435
17. Crutchield et al KE (1998) Quantitative analysis of cerebral vasculopathy in patients with Fabry disease. Neurology 50:1746–1749
18. Scott RM, Smith ER (2009) Moyamoya disease and moyamoya syndrome. N Engl J Med 19(360):1226–1237
19. Kawashima M et al (2009) Unilateral hemispheric proliferation of Ivy sign on fluid-attenuated inversion recovery images in Moyamoya disease correlates highly with ipsilateral hemispheric decrease of cerebrovascular reserve. AJNR 27
20. Suzuki J, Kodama N (1983) Moyamoya disease-a review. Stroke 14:104–109

Chapter 8
Haematological Disorders

They represent about 1 % of all types of strokes and are proportionally more frequent in young subjects.

They may present in the form of cerebral infarction, cerebral haemorrhage or cerebral venous thrombosis. There are many aetiologies: sickle-cell anaemia (infarct), myeloproliferative disorder, hereditary thrombophilias (CVT), leukaemia (haemorrhage), antiphospholipid antibodies, thrombotic thrombocytopenic purpura or thrombotic microangiopathy (recurrent TIAs), disseminated intravascular coagulation.

The clinical features and imaging of strokes associated with clotting disorders are not specific (apart from the general context: neoplasia for DIC, obstetric history or systemic inflammatory disease such as lupus for APS). The diagnosis is suspected on systematic laboratory tests (full blood count, platelets, fibrinogen, PT, APTT) or a more specific abnormality (including hereditary thrombophilia) investigated in certain cases (ischaemic stroke in young adults).

Sickle-Cell Anaemia

Pathophysiology

Autosomal recessive hereditary disease, causing an alteration of haemoglobin (haemoglobin S). Sickle-cell anaemia is the most common genetic disease in France and probably in the world (it affects 90,000 to 100,000 Americans). Haemoglobin S polymerises in the presence of hypoxia, leading to arterial or venous thromboses and red blood cell lysis. Mechanism of ischaemic strokes: vascular stenosis due to mural deposits of sickle cells in large vessel disease or vascular occlusion in small-vessel disease.

G. Saliou et al., *Practical Guide to Neurovascular Emergencies*,
DOI: 10.1007/978-2-8178-0481-1_8, © Springer-Verlag France 2014

Diagnosis

Blood smear from fresh blood: sickle-shaped or holly-leaf-shaped red blood cells.

Haemoglobin electrophoresis: single band of haemoglobin S (abnormally slow migration) if homozygous and double band of haemoglobin S (slowest) and haemoglobin A (normal) if heterozygous (healthy carrier).

Clinical Features

Various systemic clinical syndromes: vaso-occlusive crises due to arterial or venous thromboses, haemolytic anaemia and increased risk of infection (pneumococci, meningococci) secondary to repeated splenic infarcts (functional asplenia).

Neurological complications: cerebral arterial infarction or venous thrombosis. Leading cause of stroke in Afro-American children.

Characteristic involvement of the internal carotid artery bifurcation leading to moyamoya syndrome (Fig. 8.1). Possible involvement of more distal intracranial arteries (Fig. 8.2).

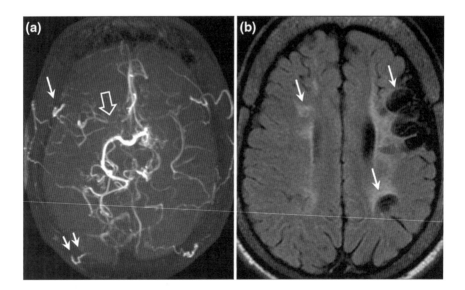

Fig. 8.1 Sickle-cell anaemia in a 26-year-old male patient resulting in moyamoya syndrome. The TOF sequence shows bilateral terminal internal carotid artery occlusion (**a** *hollow arrow*, occluded right internal carotid artery) with dural collateral vessels derived from the middle meningeal arteries (**a** *single arrow*, right middle meningeal artery) and occipital arteries (**a** *double arrows*, right occipital artery). The FLAIR sequence shows numerous ischaemic parenchymal scars (**b** *arrows*)

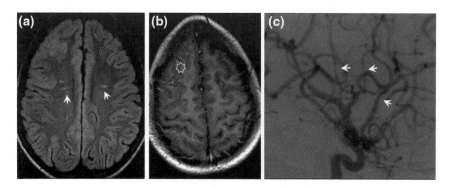

Fig. 8.2 Sickle-cell anaemia in a 12-year-old boy resulting in intracranial angiopathy. MRI signal abnormalities on the FLAIR sequence with focal white matter hyperintensities (**a** *arrows*). Right frontal pial contrast enhancement on gadolinium-enhanced T1-weighted SE sequences (**b** *star*). Arteriography shows segmental stenoses (**c** lateral view of right internal carotid artery: *arrows*)

Imaging

MRI

Moyamoya appearance: stenosis of internal carotid artery bifurcation on TOF sequence and development of choroidal and lenticulostriate collateral circulation visible on TOF sequences when the collateral circulation is well developed or on T2-weighted SE or gadolinium-enhanced T1-weighted sequences in the form of hypointensities (T2) or punctate enhanced hyperintensities (gadolinium-enhanced T1-weighted images) of the basal ganglia. More distal focal narrowing of intracranial arteries, sometimes visible on TOF sequences. Atypical sites of aneurysm sometimes visible on TOF sequences or gadolinium-enhanced T1-weighted volume-rendering images of distal vessels as intense nodular cortical enhancement.

Association of recent infarction visualized as focal hyperintensities on diffusion-weighted images with decreased ADC and old infarcts visualized as hyperintensities on FLAIR and T2-weighted images with increased ADC of the white matter or cortex predominantly adjacent to anterior watershed zones.

On T2-weighted GE images, focal hypointensities in the parenchyma or cortical sulci, sometimes visible as a result of haemorrhagic infarcts or sequelae of meningeal haemorrhage.

Angiography

Distal stenoses of internal carotid arteries with development of collateral circulation derived from anterior choroidal arteries, posterior communicating arteries and lenticulostriate arteries with the characteristic "puff of smoke" appearance. Multiple focal stenoses visible more distally in the intracranial arteries. Collateral circulation derived from the external carotid arteries (middle meningeal arteries ++) with transdural vascularization and development of the intracranial ophthalmic anastomotic network via ethmoidal arteries.

Treatment

- Hydration and oxygenation during vaso-occlusive crises. Analgesics if necessary.
- Blood transfusion and folic acid supplement to treat anaemia.
- Blood transfusion to maintain haemoglobin S level below 30 % in order to reduce the risks of stroke and arterial deposits.
- Prevention of risk factors for vaso-occlusive crisis (cold, altitude, dehydration).

Coagulopathies

Hereditary Thrombophilias

Autosomal dominant transmission.

Epidemiology

Incidence: 10 % of the population. Known risk factor for cerebral venous thrombosis. The role of hereditary thrombophilias in cerebral arterial disease remains controversial.

Aetiologies

- Activated protein C resistance due to factor V Leiden mutation (20–25 % of thrombophilias, only in Caucasian subjects).
- Prothrombin gene mutation.
- Protein C deficiency.
- Protein S deficiency.
- Congenital antithrombin III deficiency.

Acquired antithrombin deficiencies are also observed: hepatocellular failure, heparin, nephrotic syndrome and protein C or S deficiency: VKA, vitamin K deficiency, DIC, hepatocellular failure.

Neurological Indications for Investigation of Hereditary Thrombophilia

Screening for hereditary thrombophilia must not be systematic, but should be reserved for:

- patients with a history of cerebral venous thrombosis,
- young subjects treated for ischaemic stroke:
    - patients with a personal or family history of venous thrombosis and a negative aetiological work-up for ischaemic stroke,
    - or in the presence of patent foramen ovale on TOE (paradoxical embolism responsible for ischaemic stroke).

Imaging

Nonspecific signs related to venous thrombotic and haemorrhagic phenomena: venous infarctions (Fig. 8.3), subarachnoid haemorrhages and intraparenchymal haematomas.

Treatment

- Long-term effective anticoagulant therapy should be considered, depending on the type of abnormality detected (not all hereditary thrombophilias are associated with the same risk of thrombosis).
- At least: antiplatelet therapy.
- Propose family screening.

Subacute or Chronic DIC

Formation of blood clots triggered by a systemic inflammatory response induced by cytokines, leading to consumption of platelets and clotting factors. Fibrin deposits in small and medium-sized vessels leading to disseminated infarcts. DIC is secondary to an underlying disease.

Clinical Features

- Known active cancer or first sign of an underlying cancer.
- General malaise.
- Features of encephalopathy or focal deficits associated with multiple relapsing ischaemic strokes.

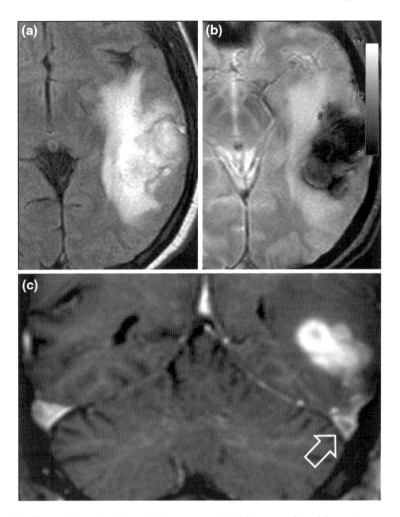

Fig. 8.3 45-year-old male patient with temporo-occipital intraparenchymal haematoma second-ary to cerebral venous thrombosis. The haematoma is hyperintense on the FLAIR sequence (**a**) and hypointense on the T2*-weighted images (**b**). The thrombus is visible in the left transverse sinus (**c** coronal gadolinium-enhanced T1-weighted images, *hollow arrow*). Laboratory tests revealed a factor II mutation and positive antiphospholipid antibodies

Laboratory Diagnosis

- Thrombocytopenia.
- Prolonged APTT.
- Decreased fibrinogen levels.
- Decreased factor V activity.
- High D-dimer levels, presence of soluble complexes (FDP).

- In chronic DIC, platelets, fibrinogen and PT can be borderline, hence the importance of **D-Dimers** and repeated laboratory tests (laboratory test results can return to normal in response to even preventive doses of heparin [LMWH]).

Imaging

Multiple, nonspecific, small cerebral infarctions (Fig. 8.4).

Associated systemic infarctions. Subarachnoid haemorrhages and intraparenchymal haematomas and sometimes intra-ocular haemorrhage may be observed.

Treatment

Treatment of the cause. Heparin can correct laboratory abnormalities but is only partially effective to prevent recurrence.

Myeloproliferative Disorders

The risk factors for arterial and venous thromboses are: age above 65 years, personal history of arterial or venous thrombosis, presence of cardiovascular risk factors.

Thromboses are the leading cause of morbidity and mortality in these diseases. Arterial thromboses are more frequent: 50–70 % of cases.

Venous thromboses are observed in 30–40 % of cases.

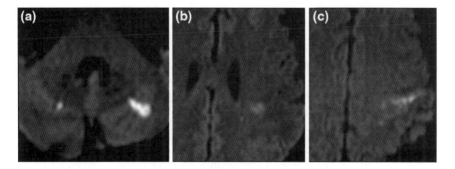

Fig. 8.4 57-year-old male patient with chronic DIC in a context of lung cancer with pancreatic, liver and bone metastases. Multiple microinfarctions affecting several vascular territories, visualized as focal hyperintensities on diffusion-weighted images (**a**, **b** and **c**)

Polycythaemia Vera (Fig. 8.5)

Pathophysiology

The annual risk of thrombosis is 4–10 %. Annual incidence of stroke or transient ischaemic attack: 4–5 %. Vascular thrombotic risk due to blood hyperviscosity (increased haematocrit) and increased thromboxane A2 synthesis, inducing platelet activation.

Risk of cerebral haemorrhage for platelet counts exceeding $1,500,000/mm^3$ and acquired Von Willebrand factor deficiency.

Clinical Features

Hyperviscosity syndrome with HBP, headache, blurred vision, tinnitus.

Diagnosis

- Haematocrit >51 % in men and >48 % in women.
- Eliminate secondary polycythaemia: chronic hypoxia, renal disease by determination of blood volume.
- Bone marrow biopsy: haematopoiesis.
- Associated with JAK-2 mutations in 95 % of cases. The thrombotic role of JAK-2 mutation is uncertain.

Treatment

- Prevention of thromboses by **antiplatelet therapy except in patients with a history of severe haemorrhage.**
- Phlebotomy to maintain haematocrit below 45 %.
- Myelosuppression using hydroxyurea.

Essential Thrombocytosis (Fig. 8.6)

Pathophysiology

Vascular complications of essential thrombocytosis are arterial thromboses in 30–40 % of cases and venous thromboses in 5 % of cases. The thrombotic risk is due to abnormal platelet behaviour with adhesion of platelets to the endothelium. Increased risk of thrombosis if platelet count $> 1,000,000/mm^3$. Frequent TIAs, sometimes pseudomigrainous.

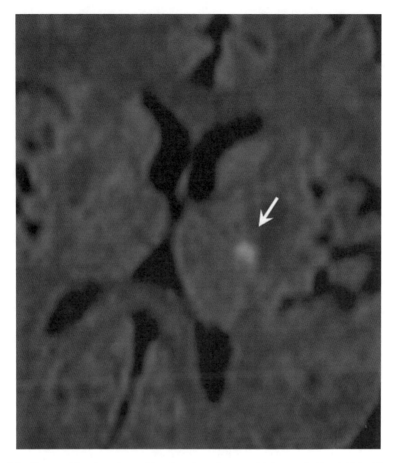

Fig. 8.5 62-year-old male patient with polycythaemia vera with haemoglobin of 15.5 g/dl. Deep focal infarct in the anterior choroidal artery territory visualized as hyperintensity on diffusion-weighted images (*arrow*)

Clinical Features

Look for disorders of the microcirculation such as erythromelalgia (present in 40 % of cases): intense pain and red, congested extremities.

Diagnosis

Platelet count > 600,000/mm^3 in the absence of inflammatory syndrome or iron deficiency, real or functional asplenia.

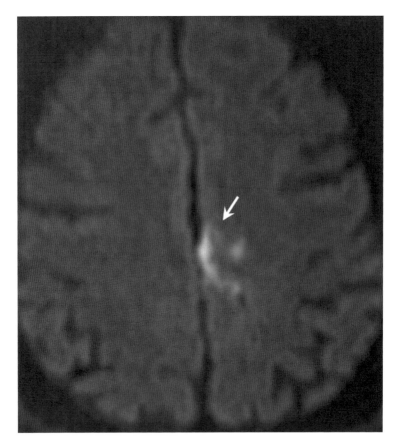

Fig. 8.6 47-year-old male patient with essential thrombocytosis, with a focal cortical infarct in the anterior cerebral artery territory visualized as hyperintensity on diffusion-weighted images (*arrow*)

Treatment

- Prevention of thromboses by **antiplatelet therapy** despite the bleeding risk.
- Hydroxyurea therapy when the platelet count > 1,500,000, age > 60 years and history of thrombosis or haemorrhage.

Antiphospholipid Syndrome (APS)

Risk factor for arterial and venous thrombosis. Stroke or TIAs are the presenting sign of APS in 20 % of cases. The risk of stroke recurrence is correlated with the level of antiphospholipid antibodies. Arterial and venous infarction associated with a prothrombotic condition caused by antibodies.

Diagnosis

APS is defined by a combination of:

- arterial or venous thrombosis and/or morbidity during pregnancy: repeated miscarriages, placental abruption, eclampsia,
- and positive antiphospholipid antibodies on two blood samples twelve weeks apart:
  - circulating lupus anticoagulant,
  - anticardiolipin antibodies,
  - beta-2-glycoprotein 1a antibodies.

Anticardiolipin antibodies are considered to be positive when >40 GPL units on two samples 3 months apart.
APS can be either primary or secondary (systemic lupus erythematosus).

Brain Imaging

Nonspecific appearance. Cerebral infarctions are usually small, multiple and situated in the subcortical white matter (Fig. 8.7).

Echocardiography

High frequency of associated nonspecific valvular heart disease (predominantly mitral valve) possibly responsible for cardioembolic stroke.

Transthoracic echocardiography reveals valvular heart disease in one-third of patients, most in the form of valvular thickening.

Treatment (HAS Guidelines [French National Authority220 for Health])

- When antiphospholipid antibodies are detected on a blood sample in a context of TIA or stroke: lifetime antiplatelet therapy.
- If TIA or stroke in the context of APS (as defined above): oral anticoagulant therapy with target INR between 2 and 3.

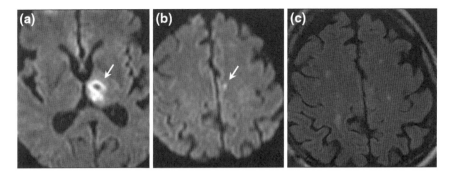

Fig. 8.7 Deep and focal cortical infarcts in two different arterial territories visualized as hyperintensities on diffusion-weighted images (**a** and **b** *arrows*). Sequelae of bilateral focal frontal white matter ischaemia visualized as focal hyperintensities on FLAIR images (**c**). Laboratory tests demonstrated the presence of anticardiolipin antibody with antinuclear factor 1/640

Thrombotic Microangiopathy (TMA) or Thrombotic Thrombocytopenic Purpura

Diagnostic emergency, rapidly fatal in 90 % of cases in the absence of treatment.

Pathophysiology

Defective cleavage of von Willebrand factor multimers by ADAMTS13 metalloprotease due to either enzyme deficiency or enzyme inactivation by autoantibodies. Von Willebrand factor circulates in the form of large multimers causing platelet activation and adhesion and the formation of multisystem arteriolar and capillary hyalin microthrombi (kidneys and brain ++). Female predominance: 3/1.

Clinical Features

- Fever, HT. Relapsing transient focal neurological deficits in 75 % of cases, seizures in 9 % of cases, encephalopathy.
- Frequent renal impairment with acute renal failure in 5 % of cases. Haemorrhagic skin lesions in 20–30 % of cases.
- Classical pentad in 20–40 % of cases: haemolytic anaemia, thrombocytopenia, neurological symptoms, fever and renal impairment.

Laboratory Diagnosis

- Haemolytic anaemia.
- Thrombocytopenia.
- Hyperbilirubinaemia, very low haptoglobin, elevated LDH.
- Blood smear: schizocytes.
- Renal failure.

Aetiologies

Idiopathic, lupus, malignant hypertension, neoplasm, infections (HIV), medications (ticlopidine, cyclosporin).

Imaging

Microvascular involvement of predominantly supratentorial white matter or grey matter: focal cortical and/or subcortical infarcts (Fig. 8.8). Infarcts are sometimes more extensive when a medium-sized artery is involved.

Intraparenchymal haemorrhages are possible but rare, predominantly supratentorial or in the brainstem.

Treatment

- Plasma exchange.
- Treatment of the cause.

Heparin-Induced Thrombocytopenia (HIT)

HIT is a rare but severe disease with an incidence of 3–5 % in patients treated by unfractionated heparin and 1 % in patients treated by LMWH.

HIT should be considered in patients treated with heparin and presenting:

– thrombocytopenia with a platelet count less than 1,00,000 and/or 30–50 % decrease in platelet count compared to baseline,
– venous or arterial thrombosis,
– heparin resistance with extension of the initial thrombotic process.

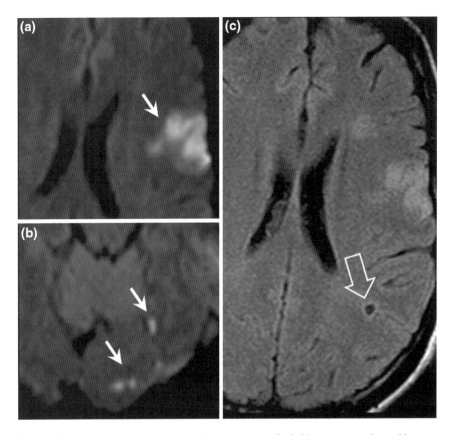

Fig. 8.8 32-year-old female patient with no pqst medical history presenting with acute neurological deficit associated with profound thrombocytopenia revealing the diagnosis of thrombotic microangiopathy. Cortical infarcts in two different arterial territories visualized as hyperintensities on diffusion-weighted images (**a** and **b** *arrows*). Sequelae from focal ischaemia visualized as a hypointense lacuna on FLAIR images (**c** *hollow arrow*)

When thrombocytopenia is observed after 5–10 days of heparin therapy, the mechanism is immunoallergic with a risk of arterial or venous (often multiple) thrombotic events.

Laboratory Diagnosis

- Platelet activation test in the presence of heparin and Orgaran® (danaparoid).
- Test for anti-heparin–platelet factor 4 complex (anti-PF4) antibodies.

Treatment

- Discontinue heparin therapy.
- Alternative antithrombotic treatment by Orgaran® (danaparoid).
- **Oral** VKA therapy until platelet count returns to baseline value, i.e. higher than 150,000.
- Life-time contraindication to heparin.

Idiopathic Hypereosinophilic Syndrome

- Unexplained major hypereosinophilia for more than 6 months associated with multiple organ dysfunction (neurological, digestive, cardiac, dermatological) secondary to eosinophilic infiltration.
- Ischaemic stroke in 12 % of cases, often multiple strokes related to the underlying heart disease.

Diagnosis

Hypereosinophilia $>1.5 \times 10^9/L$.

Treatment

Corticosteroids, tyrosine kinase inhibitors (imatinib).

Paroxysmal Nocturnal Haemoglobinuria (Marchiafava-Micheli Syndrome)

Rare disease occurring in young adults, characterized by episodes of haemolysis, often at night accompanied by "cherry red" urine.

It is the only acquired corpuscular haemolytic anaemia. CD55 and CD59-deficiency leading to red blood cell lysis when complement is activated (especially by an acidic medium, at night) and release of procoagulant substances by platelets.

It is a rare cause of cerebral venous thrombosis.

Diagnosis

- Normocytic anaemia, reticulocyte count $> 100,000/mm^3$, decreased haptoglobin, negative direct Coombs test.
- Immunophenotyping: CD55 and CD59-deficient white blood cells, red blood cells and platelets.

Treatment

- In severe forms with venous thrombosis (Budd-Chiari syndrome), aplasia, major haemolysis: allogeneic haematopoietic stem cell transplantation.
- CVT should preferably be treated by Orgaran® due to the risk of activation of affected platelets by heparin.
- Treatment by eculizumab can be considered.

Selected References

1. Lee MT et al (2006) STOP study investigators. Stroke prevention trial in sickle cell anemia (STOP): extended follow-up and final results. Blood 108:847–852
2. Roach ES et al (2008) American heart association stroke council; council on cardiovascular disease in the young. Management of stroke in infants and children: a scientific statement from a special writing group of the american heart association stroke council and the council on cardiovascular disease in the young. Stroke 39:2644–2691
3. Oguz KK et al (2003) Sickle cell disease: continuous arterial spin-labeling perfusion MR imaging in children. Radiology 227:567–574
4. Hart RG, Kanter MC (1990) Hematologic disorders and ischemic stroke A selective review. Stroke 21:1111–1121
5. Martinez HR et al (1993) Ischemic stroke due to deficiency of coagulation inhibitors. Report of 10 young adults. Stroke 24:19–25
6. Landolfi R et al (2004) Efficacy and safety of low-dose aspirin in polycythemia vera. N Engl J Med 350:114–124
7. Levine SR et al (2004) Antiphospholipid antibodies and subsequent thrombo-occlusive events in patients with ischemic stroke. JAMA 291:576–584
8. Keeling D et al. (2012) British Committee for Standards in Haematology. Guidelines on the investigation and management of antiphospholipid syndrome. Br J Haematol 157(1):47–58
9. Bousser MG, Mas JL (2009)Traité de neurologie. Accident vasculaire cérébraux. Edition Dion 711–725

Chapter 9
Cerebral Haemorrhage

Intraparenchymal Haemorrhage

The most serious form of stroke: 1-month mortality = 40 %.

Definition

Intraparenchymal haemorrhage due to rupture of small vessels. May rupture into the ventricles. Usually not associated with subarachnoid haemorrhage.

Clinical Features

Sudden onset of neurological deficit ± headache. There is no clinical criterion to differentiate between haemorrhage and infarction.

Aetiologies

- Vascular causes: high blood pressure (leading cause) (Figs. 9.1 and 9.2), cerebral amyloid angiopathy (Fig. 9.3), cerebral vasculitis, cerebral venous thrombosis, cerebral arteriovenous malformation (Fig. 9.4), dural fistula, aneurysm (rare in the case of isolated cerebral haemorrhage without meningeal haemorrhage), cavernous malformation, haemorrhagic transformation of infarction.
- Non-vascular causes: clotting disorders (leukaemia, anticoagulant or antiplatelet therapy), primary (Fig. 9.5) and secondary brain tumours.

G. Saliou et al., *Practical Guide to Neurovascular Emergencies*,
DOI: 10.1007/978-2-8178-0481-1_9, © Springer-Verlag France 2014

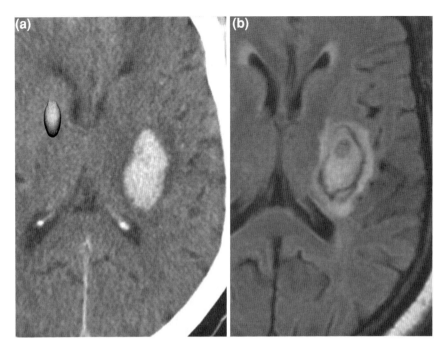

Fig. 9.1 Very acute phase of intraparenchymal haemorrhage of the posterior limb of the left internal capsule (oxyhaemoglobin) occurring during a hypertensive crisis. The haematoma is hyperdense (**a**) on CT scan and hyperintense on the MRI FLAIR sequence (**b**). The site of the haematoma in the posterior limb of the internal capsule is characteristic of haematomas due to hypertensive crisis

Aetiological Work-Up

- Look for HBP (not always known before onset of haemorrhage).
- Look for predisposing laboratory abnormalities:

  – Complete blood count, platelets, PT, APTT, thrombin time.

- Systematic ECG.
- Look for complications of HBP: TTE (left ventricular hypertrophy), renal function, funduscopy.
- When the site of the haematoma is unusual for HBP (although haematomas associated with HBP can occur anywhere), or in the absence of HBP or multiple haematomas and when the clinical features are suggestive: investigations to detect underlying neoplasm (chest, abdomen, pelvis CT scan).
- Three months after the acute episode, brain MRI must be systematically performed to detect an underlying lesion (tumour or vascular [cavernous malformation or arteriovenous malformation]) that may have been initially masked by blood or compressed by the haematoma.

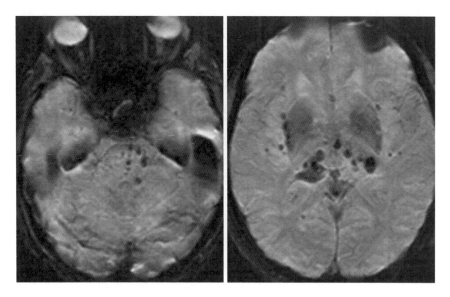

Fig. 9.2 Patient with a history of chronic hypertension. Multiple deep intraparenchymal microhaemorrhages visualized as focal hypointensities involving the brainstem and basal ganglia on T2*-weighted images

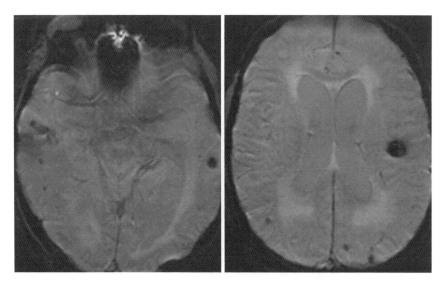

Fig. 9.3 Patient with cerebral amyloid angiopathy. Multiple peripheral cortico-subcortical intraparenchymal microhaemorrhages visualized as focal hypointensities on T2*-weighted images

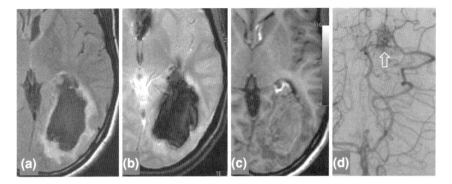

Fig. 9.4 Acute phase of left occipital intraparenchymal haemorrhage (deoxyhaemoglobin). The haematoma is hypointense with a hyperintense corona on the FLAIR sequence (**a**), hypointense on T2*-weighted images (**b**) and isointense on T1-weighted images (**c**). Arteriography shows an arteriovenous malformation responsible for bleeding (**d** *hollow arrow*)

Imaging

CT

Hyperdense intraparenchymal collection. Hypodensity around the lesion associated with resorption of oedema or mass effect. Usual site in basal ganglia in the case of HBP. However, the site of the haematoma is not predictive of the cause. CSF-blood fluid level (hypodense-hyperdense fluid level) in the case of intraventricular haemorrhage.

MRI

- Signal varies with time (Table 9.1).
- May be associated with other old haematomas visualized as hypointensity on T2-weighted gradient-echo images.
- AVM: evidence of flow voids over the haematoma.
- Definitive diagnosis: venous arterialization on TOF sequences. Perfusion-weighted imaging: marked increase in CBV and decreased MTT over the AVM.

Treatment

Treatment of the cause. Blood pressure control (target values during the acute phase of haemorrhage: systolic BP: 180 mmHg, diastolic BP: 90 mmHg).

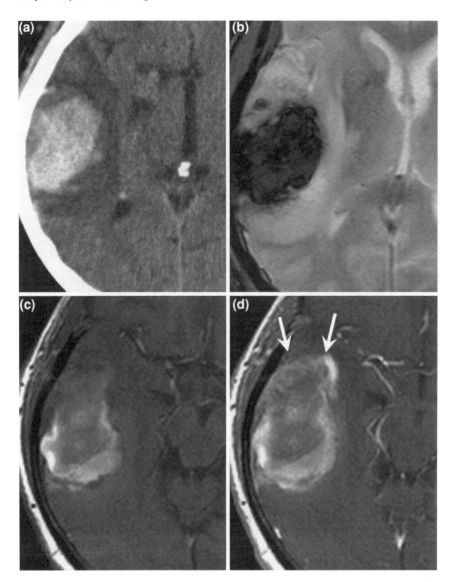

Fig. 9.5 Right temporal intraparenchymal haemorrhage secondary to brain tumour. The haematoma is hyperdense on CT scan (**a**), hypointense on T2*-weighted images (**b**) and heterogeneous (hyper- and iso-intense) on T1-weighted images (**c**). Note the anterior nodular contrast enhancement (**d** gadolinium-enhanced T1-weighted sequence, *arrows*), which raised the suspicion of an underlying lesion. Postoperative histological examination demonstrated glioblastoma

Table 9.1 CT and MRI appearance of haematomas according to the stage of haemoglobin degradation and over time

Stage	hemoglobin degradation	Density on CT-scan	Signal intensity on MR		
			SE T1	SE T2/Flair	T2*
Hyperacute (0-3h)	*OxyHb*	Iso/hyper	Iso	Hyper	Rim hypo
Acute (4h-3d)	*DesoxyHb*	Hyper	Iso	Center hypo Rim hyper	Hypo
Early subacute (4d-7d)	*MetHb Intra*	Hyper/iso	Center iso Rim hyper	Hypo	Hypo
Late subacute (1w-4w)	*MetHb Extra*	Iso/hypo	Hyper	Hyper	Rim hypo
Chronic (>1 month)	*Hemosidérine*	Hypo	Hypo/Iso/hyper	Hypo/iso/hyper	Rim hypo

Anticoagulants and antiplatelet agents are contraindicated. The only exception is cerebral venous thrombosis, in which anticoagulants are the mainstay of treatment.

Meningeal Haemorrhage

Until proved otherwise, any nontraumatic meningeal haemorrhage is due to ruptured intracranial aneurysm!

When an aneurysm is discovered, always look for one or more other aneurysms (multiple aneurysms in 20 % of patients).

Subarachnoid haemorrhage between arachnoid and pia mater.

Clinical Features

Typically sudden thunderclap headache, but can be less severe and more progressive. Meningeal syndrome with neck stiffness and photophobia. Impairment of consciousness or coma. Mortality rate: 30 % in the acute phase and 50 % in the first month if haemorrhage is associated with ruptured intracranial aneurysm.

The aetiology can be suggested by the site of bleeding:

- Lateral sulcus: aneurysm at the middle cerebral artery bifurcation;
- Frontal interhemispheric: aneurysm of the anterior communicating artery or pericallosal artery;
- Basal cistern: aneurysm of the posterior communicating artery;
- Posterior fossa: aneurysm of the vertebrobasilar system;
- Exclusively perimesencephalic: no known aetiology in 90 % of cases.

Aetiologies

- Rupture of intracranial aneurysm (80 % of cases), often profuse haemorrhage in the lateral sulcus and basal cisterns (Fig. 9.6).
- Head injury.
- Cerebral vasculitis, reversible cerebral vasoconstriction syndrome, cerebral amyloid angiopathy.
- Intracranial arterial dissection.
- Idiopathic (particularly in perimesencephalic haemorrhage).

When focal meningeal haemorrhage involves the convexity away from the cisterns and the lateral sulci, four main aetiologies: cerebral amyloid angiopathy (Fig. 9.7), cortical venous thrombosis, reversible cerebral vasoconstriction syndrome and cerebral vasculitis.

Imaging

Classification of meningeal haemorrhages due to ruptured aneurysm according to Fischer:

- grade 1: haemorrhage not visible on imaging (diagnosed by lumbar puncture);
- grade 2: subarachnoid haemorrhage less than 1 mm thick;
- grade 3: subarachnoid haemorrhage more than 1 mm thick;
- grade 4: subarachnoid haemorrhage in combination with intraparenchymal haemorrhage or intraventricular haemorrhage.

CT

CT can sometimes be normal: lumbar puncture must be performed to exclude meningeal haemorrhage.

CT is the standard procedure to detect meningeal haemorrhage.

Hyperdensity of one or more cortical sulci and/or basal cisterns.

Brain CT angiography may demonstrate an aneurysm responsible for the haemorrhage.

MRI

Haemorrhage in cortical sulci is hyperintense on T2-weighted SE images and FLAIR images and hypointense on T2*-weighted images. An aneurysm may be visualized on the TOF sequence.

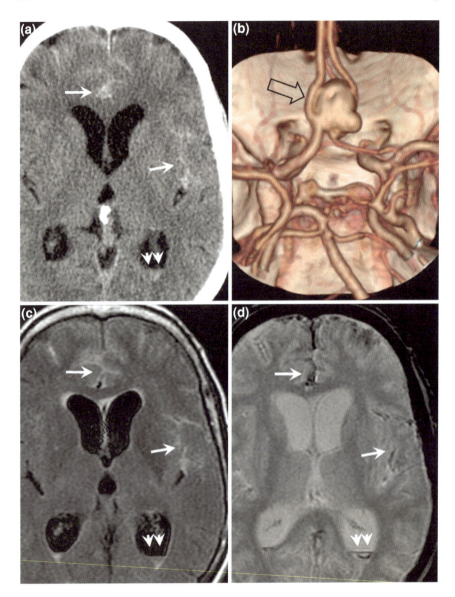

Fig. 9.6 Ruptured intracranial aneurysm with Fischer grade 4 subarachnoid meningeal haemorrhage in a 57-year-old female patient. CT visualizes the haemorrhage as hyperdensities of cortical sulci, well seen in the interhemispheric region and left lateral sulcus (**a** *simple arrows*). There is an associated intraventricular haemorrhage visualized as a fluid level in the occipital horns (**a** *double arrows*). CT angiography shows ruptured aneurysm of the anterior communicating artery (**b** *hollow arrow*). On MRI, the haemorrhage is hyperintense on the FLAIR sequence (**c**) and hypointense on T2*-weighted images (**d**)

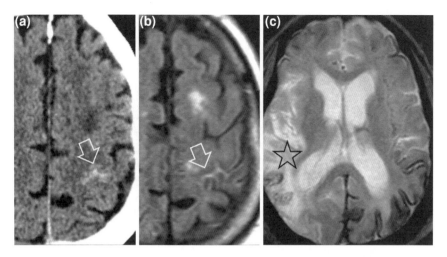

Fig. 9.7 70-year-old patient with focal meningeal haemorrhage hyperdense on CT (**a** *hollow arrow*) and hyperintense on MRI FLAIR sequence (**b** *hollow arrow*). Cognitive decline for several years, not investigated. Cerebral amyloid angiopathy was diagnosed on the basis of the clinical features and associated chronic lesions discovered on MRI: areas of cortical gliosis (**c** *star*) and diffuse superficial siderosis reflecting chronic meningeal haemorrhages visualized as cortical hypointensity on T2*-weighted images (**c**)

Arteriography

- Standard procedure to demonstrate intracranial aneurysm or cerebral vasculitis.
- Localization:
  - Internal carotid artery in 30 % of patients (particularly origin of posterior communicating artery and origin of anterior choroidal artery);
  - Anterior communicating artery in 30 % of patients;
  - Middle cerebral artery in 20 % of patients (particularly middle cerebral artery bifurcation);
  - Vertebrobasilar system in 10 % of patients (particularly origin of PICA and terminal segment of basilar artery).

Treatment

Embolization by coils or emergency surgical treatment by clip if aneurysm (risk of "re-rupture" and clinical deterioration of patient if treatment delayed). Indications depend on the size of the aneurysm, the size of the neck and its site. First-line endovascular treatment is often indicated.

Cerebral Amyloid Angiopathy (Fig. 9.8)

Definition

Chronic intracranial small artery disease, particularly cortical.

Amyloid protein deposition in the media and adventitia of cortical arterioles and capillaries. Common cause of recurrent cortical haemorrhages of the elderly. Sporadic forms are more frequent.

Hereditary forms are very rare and varied (many genes identified).

Clinical Features

Acute presentation if lobar haematoma. A chronic presentation in the form of dementia is also possible. Incidence: 50 % after the age of 80. Accounts for 10 to 15 % of cerebral haemorrhages after the age of 60.

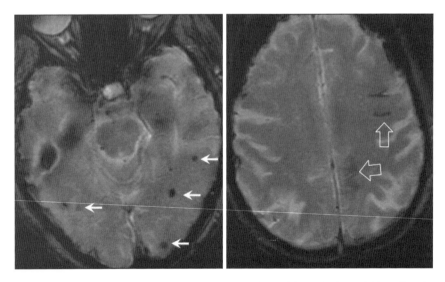

Fig. 9.8 MRI T2* sequence (gradient-echo) in a patient with cerebral amyloid angiopathy. Multiple microhaemorrhages visualized as predominantly cortical and subcortical hypointensities (*simple arrows*). Associated subarachnoid gyriform hypointensities related to old meningeal haemorrhages (*hollow arrows*)

Diagnosis

Boston criteria:

1. Definite cerebral amyloid angiopathy (post mortem examination of the brain): lobar, cortical or cortical/subcortical haemorrhage + severe cerebral amyloid angiopathy + no other aetiology.
2. Probable cerebral amyloid angiopathy with supporting pathological evidence (evacuated haematoma or cortical biopsy): lobar, cortical or cortical/subcortical haemorrhage, + vascular amyloid deposition + no other aetiology.
3. Probable cerebral amyloid angiopathy (post mortem = 100 %): multiple lobar, cortical or cortical/subcortical (including cerebellum) haemorrhages (including microhaemorrhages) + age $\geq$ 55 years + no other aetiology.
4. Possible cerebral amyloid angiopathy (post mortem = 60 %): single lobar, cortical or cortical/subcortical haemorrhage + age $\geq$ 55 years + no other aetiology.

Imaging

CT

Lobar haematoma (especially frontal lobe haematoma) with spontaneous cortical or subcorticalhyperdensity, not involving the basal ganglia (in contrast with haemorrhage secondary to HBP). Associated areas of cerebral ischaemia within the cortical territory. Gyriform calcifications, sequelae of old haemorrhages. Leukoaraiosis

MRI

Variable signal depending on the age of the lobar haematoma (Table 9.1). Areas of cortical ischaemia. Multiple microhaemorrhages (microbleeds) visualized as cortical/subcortical hypointensities on T2*-weighted images. Gyriform hypointensities (siderosis) on T2*-weighted images, sometimes isolated, associated with old cortical subarachnoid haemorrhages.

A pseudoneoplastic appearance may be rarely observed (Fig. 9.9) with mass effect and possible cerebromeningeal contrast enhancement.

Treatment

No aetiological treatment.

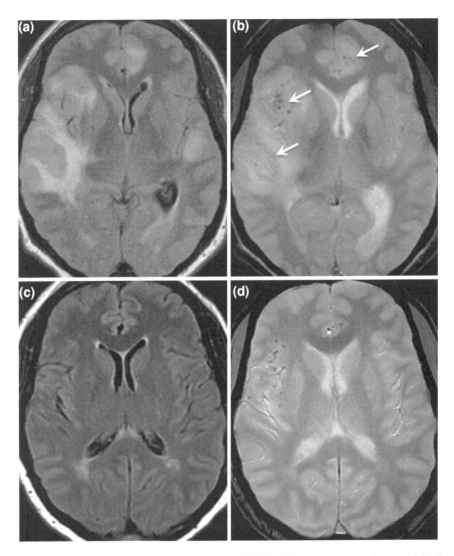

Fig. 9.9 Pseudoneoplastic amyloid angiopathy on MRI FLAIR sequence (**a**) and T2*-weighted images (**b**). Multiple hyperintense areas causing mass effect on adjacent cerebral parenchyma with slight midline shift, collapse of right lateral ventricle and loss of cortical sulci. Note the punctate hypointense microhaemorrhages within the oedema (**b** *arrows*). MR angiography and arteriography confirmed the absence of cerebral venous thrombosis which is the main differential diagnosis in this setting. Progressive resolution of symptoms in response to steroid therapy and marked reduction of MRI anomalies 3 months later

Elimination of treatments predisposing to bleeding (antiplatelet agents, anticoagulants).

Control of associated cardiovascular risk factors.

Steroid therapy can be considered in pseudoneoplastic cases.

Intracranial Cavernous Malformations

Clinical Features

Seizures (most common symptom: 40–50 % of patients), focal neurological deficit (15–45 % of patients), acute headache and/or sudden neurological deficit in the case of haematoma.

Two forms of cavernous malformations have been described: sporadic form (70 % of patients, often single lesion) and familial form (30 % of patients, often multiple lesions). If familial, autosomal dominant transmission (many genes identified). Very serious when the cavernous malformation is situated in the brainstem. Brain radiation therapy can induce the formation of cavernous malformation.

Frequently associated with a developmental venous anomaly (DVA), which must be systematically investigated by gadolinium-enhanced T1-weighted volume-rendering sequence.

Imaging

MRI classification according to Zabramski:

- Type 1 (Fig. 9.10): acute or subacute haemorrhage. Hyperintense on T1-weighted images, hyperintense or hypointense on T2-weighted SE images and hypointense on T2*-weighted images.
- Type 2 (Fig. 9.11): haemorrhages and thromboses of varying age. Reticulated or characteristic "popcorn" appearance. Mixed signal on T1-weighted images and T2-weighted SE images with hypointense rim and hypointense signal on T2*-weighted images.
- Type 3 (Fig. 9.12): chronic haemorrhage. Homogeneous hypointensity on T1-weighted images, T2-weighted SE images and T2*-weighted images.
- Type 4 (Fig. 9.13): microhaemorrhages visible on T2*-weighted images only. Barely visible or not visible on T1-weighted images and T2-weighted SE images. Multiple, punctate hypointense lesions on T2*-weighted images.

Treatment

Surgical resection of symptomatic cavernous malformations can be considered. Stereotactic radiosurgery is under evaluation. In the case of conservative management: annual follow-up MRI or in the case of new symptoms.

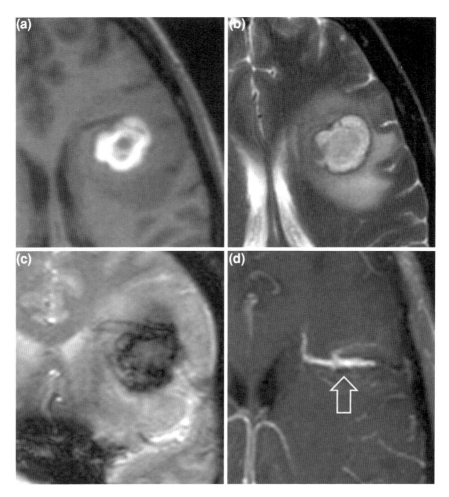

Fig. 9.10 Type 1 cavernous malformation according to Zabramski's classification (recent haemorrhage). The lesion is hyperintense on T1-weighted images (**a**), hyperintense on T2-weighted SE images (**b** *arrow*) and hypointense on T2*-weighted images (**c** coronal section). Note the associated developmental venous anomaly, well visible on the gadolinium-enhanced T1 volume-rendering sequence (**d**)

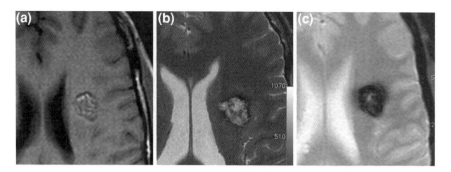

Fig. 9.11 Type 2 cavernous malformation according to Zabramski's classification. The lesion has a mixed signal on T1-weighted images (**a**), hyperintense with hypointense rim on T2-weighted SE images (**b**) and hypointense on T2*-weighted images (**c**)

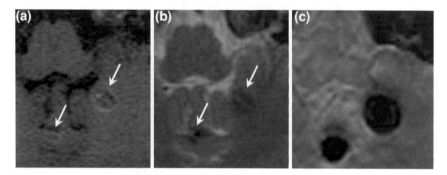

Fig. 9.12 Type 3 cavernous malformations according to Zabramski's classification. The lesions are hypointense on T1-weighted images (**a** arrows), T2-weighted SE images (**b** arrows) and T2*-weighted images (**c**). Note that the lesions are more clearly visualized on T2*-weighted images because this sequence is more sensitive to magnetic susceptibility artefacts

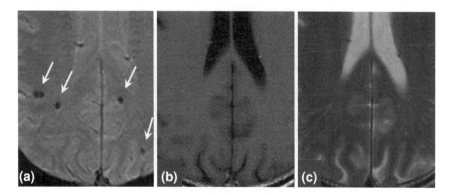

Fig. 9.13 Multiple Type 4 cavernous malformations according to Zabramski's classification (microhaemorrhages). The lesions are hypointense on T2* sequence (**a** *arrows*) and not visualized on T1 (**b**) and T2 SE sequences (**c**)

Siderosis Due to Recurrent Subarachnoid Haemorrhages (Fig. 9.14)

Superficial Siderosis is a Consequence, not a Cause!

Haemorrhage is not visible on the other sequences, particularly on FLAIR images (b). In this patient, the cause was a cauda equina paraganglioma responsible for recurrent subarachnoid meningeal haemorrhages leading to chronic haemosiderin deposits on the surface of the neuraxis.

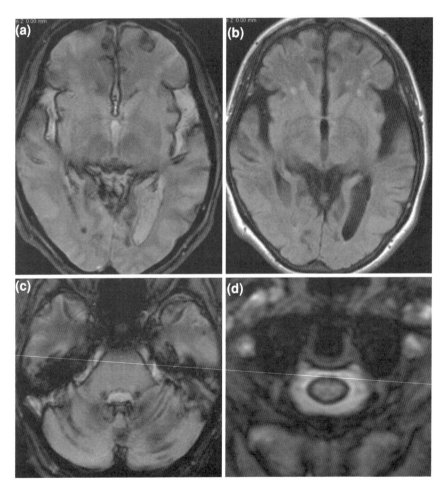

Fig. 9.14 Superficial cerebral and spinal cord siderosis in a 61-year-old female patient with early dementia and bilateral hearing loss. MRI T2*-weighted images (**a**, **c** and **d**) show a hypointense fine band on the surface of the cortex

Definition

Leptomeningeal haemosiderin deposits on the surface of the neuraxis (brain, cerebellum and brainstem, cranial nerves, spinal cord) due to chronic and/or recurrent subarachnoid haemorrhage.

Clinical Features

Progressive onset of symptoms. Cranial nerve involvement (hearing loss due to vestibulocochlear nerve lesion in 95 % of patients), cerebellar ataxia (88 %), pyramidal lesion (75 %), myelopathy, dementia. The extent of the deposits is not correlated with clinical severity. Frequently asymptomatic.

CSF is abnormal in three quarters of patients: xanthochromic or haemorrhagic CSF, elevated CSF protein, presence of siderophages, elevated ferritin.

Aetiologies

All aetiologies responsible for recurrent subarachnoid haemorrhage. No aetiology found in one half of patients (the whole neuraxis must be studied).

Brain

- Dural fistula.
- Cerebral amyloid angiopathy.
- Aneurysm.
- Tumour.
- Cavernous malformation.

Spinal Cord

- Cavernous malformation.
- Ependymoma.
- Paraganglioma of filum terminale.
- Traumatic nerve root avulsion.

Imaging

CT

Not visible. Sometimes, slightly hyperdense appearance of a cortical sulcus.
  Parenchymal atrophy is sometimes observed

MRI

Very hypointense fine band (black) on T2-weighted sequences (more prominent on
T2*-weighted images than on T2-weighted SE images). Poorly visible or not
visible on the other sequences. Sometimes slightly hyperintense on T1-weighted
sequences. Anomalies are predominantly observed in the posterior fossa: brainstem, cerebellar hemispheres and vermis, basal cisterns and cranial nerves (facial
and vestibulocochlear nerves and trigeminal nerves).

Treatment

- Treatment of the cause. No treatment for haemosiderin deposits.

Selected References

1. Grossman RI, Gomori JM, Goldberg HI, Hackney DB, Atlas SW, Kemp SS, Zimmerman
   RA, Bilaniuk LT (1988) MR imaging of hemorrhagic conditions of the head and neck.
   Radiographics 8:441–454
2. Parizel PM, Makkat S, Van Miert E, Van Goethem JW, van den Hauwe L, De Schepper AM
   (2001) Intracranial hemorrhage: principles of CT and MRI interpretation. Eur Radiol
   11:1770–1783
3. Molyneux A et al (2002) International subarachnoid aneurysm trial (ISAT) collaborative
   group. International subarachnoid aneurysm trial (ISAT) of neurosurgical clipping versus
   endovascular coiling in 2143 patients with ruptured intracranial aneurysms: a randomised
   trial. Lancet 26(360)1267–1274
4. Imaizumi T et al (2003) Detection of hemosiderin deposition by T2*-weighted MRI after
   subarachnoid hemorrhage. Stroke 34:1693–1698
5. Fiebach JB et al (2004) MRI in acute subarachnoid haemorrhage; findings with a standardised
   stroke protocol. Neuroradiology 46:44–48
6. Kumar S et al (2010) Atraumatic convexal subarachnoid hemorrhage: clinical presentation,
   imaging patterns, and etiologies. Neurology 16(74):893–899
7. Hendricks HT et al (1990) Cerebral amyloid angiopathy: diagnosis by MRI and brain biopsy.
   Neurology 40:1308–1310
8. Osumi AK et al (1995) Cerebral amyloid angiopathy presenting as a brain mass. AJNR
   16:911–915

9. Morton-Bours EC et al (1999) Cerebral amyloid angiopathy with unilateral hemorrhages, mass effect, and meningeal enhancement. Neurology 53:233–234

10. Koennecke HC (2006) Cerebral microbleeds on MRI: prevalence, associations, and potential clinical implications. Neurology 66:165–171

11. Chao CP et al (2006) Cerebral amyloid angiopathy: CT and MR imaging findings. Radiographics 26:1517–1531

12. Zabramski JM et al (1994) The natural history of familial cavernous malformations: results of an ongoing study. J Neurosurg 80:422–432

13. Brunereau L et al (2000) Familial form of intracranial cavernous angioma: MR imaging findings in 51 families. French society of neurosurgery. Radiology 214:209–216

14. Al-Shahi Salman R et al (2008) Angioma alliance scientific advisory board. Hemorrhage from cavernous malformations of the brain: definition and reporting standards. Angioma alliance scientific advisory board. Stroke 39:32

15. Kumar N et al (2006) Superficial siderosis. Neurology 66/67:1144–1152/1528

16. van Harskamp NJ et al (2005) Cognitive and social impairments in patients with superficial siderosis. Brain 128:1082–1092

17. Fearnley JM et al (1995) Superficial siderosis of the central nervous system. Brain 118:1051–1066

18. Bracchi M et al (1993) Superficial siderosis of the CNS: MR diagnosis and clinical findings. AJNR 14:227–236

Chapter 10
Cerebral Venous Thrombosis

Cerebral haemorrhage and subarachnoid haemorrhage secondary to cerebral venous thrombosis are treated by anticoagulants.

Definition

Thrombosis of a deep cerebral vein (Fig. 10.1) or a superficial cerebral vein or dural venous sinus (Fig. 10.2), generally responsible for vasogenic oedema in a venous territory (possibly associated with cytotoxic oedema) and often intraparenchymal haematoma. N.B.: venous territories are different from arterial territories and are very variable.

Clinical Features

- Incidence: 0.5 % of strokes.
- Occurs at any age with a female predominance.
- No clearly defined anatomical and clinical syndrome due to the anatomical variability of the cerebral venous system and the possible presence of collateral vessels.
- Variable onset. Classical clinical presentations: isolated intracranial hypertension (25 %) with progressive headache (always present), bilateral papilloedema on funduscopy, sometimes sixth cranial nerve palsy, shifting focal neurological deficits, seizures, disturbances of consciousness, signs of encephalopathy.
- Ten to 20 % of patients present signs of confusion or isolated psychiatric disorders or sometimes recent isolated headache with normal brain CT scan and CSF analysis.

G. Saliou et al., *Practical Guide to Neurovascular Emergencies*,
DOI: 10.1007/978-2-8178-0481-1_10, © Springer-Verlag France 2014

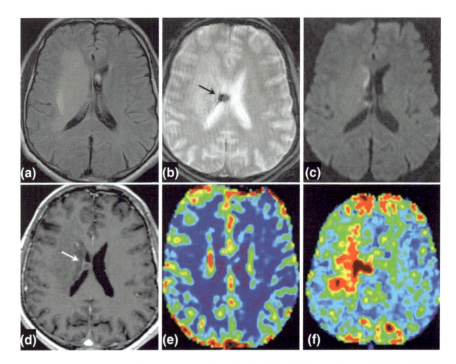

Fig. 10.1 Acute phase of deep venous thrombosis (right thalamostriate vein). The FLAIR sequence (**a**) shows the venous infarction with very limited hyperintensity on diffusion-weighted images (**c**) related to predominantly vasogenic oedema. The thrombus is visible as hypointensity on T2-weighted GE images (**b** *black arrow*) in the wall of the right lateral ventricle, with a delta sign on gadolinium-enhanced T1-weighted images (**d** *white arrow*) associated with enhancement of the vein wall without enhancement of the thrombus. The CBV (**e**) is slightly modified in the affected territory, with prolonged MTT (**f**) related to venous oedema

Aetiologies

Multiple causes are often associated.

- Local: head injury, tumours, arteriovenous malformations, developmental venous anomaly (rare).
- Infections: local (ENT: sphenoid and petrous part of temporal bone) or systemic.
- Systemic diseases: systemic lupus erythematosus, Behçet's disease, congenital thrombophilias, coagulopathies, neoplasms, haematological diseases, iron deficiency, drugs.
- Gynaecological and obstetric: postpartum more often than pregnancy and oral contraception.
- Idiopathic.

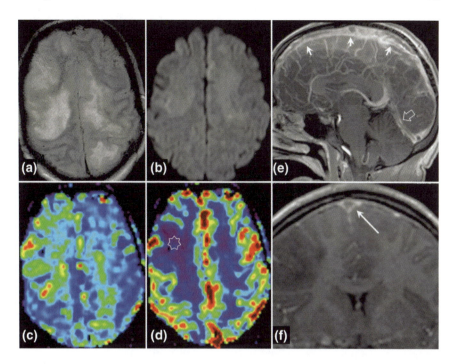

Fig. 10.2 Acute phase of cerebral venous thrombosis (superior sagittal sinus and straight sinus). Venous infarction is visible as a hyperintensity on FLAIR images (**a**) with variable signal on diffusion-weighted images (**b** ADC mainly normal or increased). Characteristic appearance of venous oedema on perfusion-weighted sequences with prolonged MTT (**c** *green and red*) compared with normal cerebral parenchyma (*blue*) and moderately decreased CBV (**d** *star*). On gadolinium-enhanced T1-weighted sequence sagittal section, thrombus is visible in the superior sagittal sinus (**e** *3 small arrows*) and straight sinus (**e** *hollow arrow*). Note the delta sign on the gadolinium-enhanced T1-weighted sequence with coronal reconstruction (**f** *long arrow*)

Investigations

- D-Dimers: if normal, excludes the diagnosis of recent venous thrombosis *except* when the patient reports isolated headache: 25 % of patients with normal D-Dimers.
- Complete blood count, platelets (looking for haematological diseases), PT, APTT, CRP.
- Lumbar puncture if feasible (meningitis, assessment of CSF pressure), before starting anticoagulant therapy. In the absence of an intracerebral lesion responsible for a mass effect, lumbar puncture is indicated in this context (even in the presence of intracranial hypertension).
- Work-up for thrombophilia: protein C, protein S, factor V Leiden, antithrombin III, prothrombin G20210A mutation, search for circulating anticoagulant,

antiβ2GP1 antibodies, anticardiolipin antibodies, antiphospholipid antibodies, antinuclear factor.
- Look for a local (especially head and neck) or systemic infectious cause or underlying neoplasm.

Imaging

Diagnosis = visualization of venous thrombosis. Absence of arterial distribution of cerebral parenchymal abnormalities.

Imaging of Veins

CT

Spontaneous hyperdensity of blood clot in a venous sinus or cerebral vein. On contrast-enhanced CT, delta sign associated with enhancement of the wall of the venous sinus, without central enhancement of the blood clot.

The walls of the venous sinus become convex due to the intraluminal thrombus.

MRI

Hyperintensity in a sinus (coronal section of the superior sagittal sinus) on T1-weighted images and T2-weighted SE images. No venous intravascular signal on phase-contrast sequences. No intravascular enhancement or mural enhancement after gadolinium injection (delta sign).

T2 GE sequences very useful to demonstrate signs of cortical venous thrombosis visualized as hypointensity in a vein.

Cerebral Parenchymal Imaging

Normal in one third of cases!

CT

Oedematous parenchymal hypodensity with effacement of cortical sulci and mass effect on adjacent structures. N.B.: thromboses of midline veins and venous sinuses can lead to bilateral lesions of the cerebral parenchyma.

Hyperdense lesion due to associated haematoma in 10–50 % of cases. Sometimes, small, isolated, focal, hyperdense meningeal haemorrhage of a cortical sulcus (Fig. 10.3).

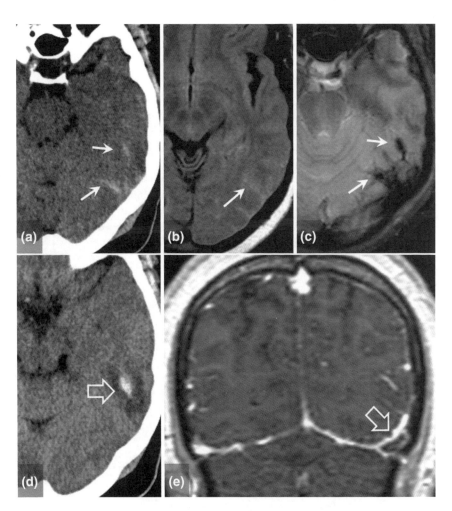

Fig. 10.3 Subarachnoid haemorrhage due to superficial venous thrombosis of the transverse sinus. Haemorrhage is hyperdense on CT scan (**a** *arrows*), hyperintense on MRI FLAIR sequences (**b** *arrow*) and hypointense on T2* sequences (**c** *arrows*). It is associated with minimal hyperdense cortical haematoma on CT (**d** *hollow arrow*). Thrombus is visible on the coronal gadolinium-enhanced T1-weighted sequence (**e** *hollow arrow*)

MRI

MRI is mainly useful to eliminate other diagnoses.

Parenchyma is hyperintense on FLAIR images, usually with heterogeneous diffusion and variable ADC (decreased with cytotoxic oedema, normal or increased with vasogenic oedema). Hyperintensity on T1-weighted images and hypointensity on T2-weighted GE images associated with parenchymal haematoma.

Treatment

Urgent!

- Antithrombotic treatment by unfractionated heparin (target APTT between 2 and 3 times control values) or low-dose LMWH, even in the presence of parenchymal haematoma. Administration of oral anticoagulants as soon as possible (target INR between 2 and 3).
- A surgical decompression flap (Fig. 10.4) can sometimes be indicated (<5 % of cases) in the case of a malignant course (very large parenchymal lesion(s)) with mass effect and clinical and/or radiological signs of uncal herniation) and remains possible even in patients with fixed dilated pupils (different outcome from that of arterial infarction with a better prognosis).
- Treatment of the cause when identified.

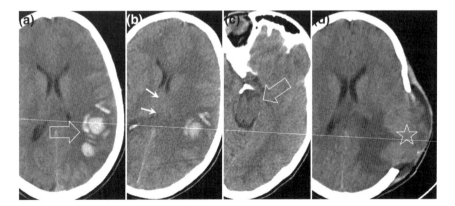

Fig. 10.4 Brain CT scan on D0 in a 20-year-old female patient with cortical haematoma (**a** *hollow arrow*, hyperdensity) associated with venous thrombosis of the superior sagittal sinus. After 24 h (**b** and **c**), increased mass effect with effacement of left lateral ventricle, onset of right subfalcine herniation (**b** *double arrows*) and left uncal herniation (**c** *hollow arrow*) constituting an indication for surgical decompression. Resolution of signs of herniation after decompression craniotomy (**d** *star*)

- Symptomatic treatments: analgesics, lumbar drain (±acetazolamide) if intracranial hypertension (in the absence of mass effect and signs of herniation), antiepileptic drugs if seizures.
- Discontinuation and contraindication of combined oestrogen-progestogen oral contraceptives and hormone replacement therapy for menopause.
- Functional and vital prognosis significantly better than that of ischaemic strokes. Mortality: 5 %, recovery without sequelae >75 %.

Selected References

1. Ferro JM et al (2004) ISCVT investigators. Prognosis of cerebral vein and dural sinus thrombosis: results of the international study on cerebral vein and dural sinus thrombosis (ISCVT). Stroke 35:664–670
2. Girot M et al (2007) ISCVT investigators. Predictors of outcome in patients with cerebral venous thrombosis and intracerebral hemorrhage. Stroke 38:337–342
3. Canhão P et al (2005) ISCVT investigators. Causes and predictors of death in cerebral venous thrombosis. Stroke 36:1720–1725
4. Einhäupl K et al (2006) EFNS guideline on the treatment of cerebral venous and sinus thrombosis. Eur J Neurol 13:553–559
5. Théaudin M et al (2010) Should decompressive surgery be performed in malignant cerebral venous thrombosis? A series of 12 patients. Stroke 25
6. Bousser MG, Mas JL (2009) Traité de neurologie. Accident vasculaire cérébraux. Ed Dion 593–613

Chapter 11
Spinal Cord Infarction

Anatomy (Fig. 11.1)

Blood supply to the spinal cord is derived from a midline anterior spinal artery and two more lateral posterior spinal arteries. Spinal cord ischaemia is generally due to a lesion of the anterior spinal artery, very rarely of a posterior spinal artery. Blood supply to the middle part of the spinal cord is derived from the anterior spinal artery. This artery is supplied by 4–8 radiculomedullary arteries derived from cervical vertebral, thoracic intercostal and lumbar arteries. The largest one is known as the artery of Adamkiewicz, generally arising on the left side at T8–T10. The posterior spinal arteries supply the peripheral region of the spinal cord and form a perispinal anastomotic pial network. These arteries are derived from 10 to 20 radiculopial arteries, branches of cervical vertebral arteries, thoracic intercostal arteries and lumbar arteries.

Pathophysiology

Two types of spinal cord infarction are distinguished:

- Global ischaemia secondary to low cardiac output (cardiac arrest, severe hypotension in a context of shock, etc.). In this case, ischaemia predominantly affects the grey matter (central region) and thoracolumbar territory (less vascularized zones);
- Focal ischaemia in the territory of an artery supplying the spinal cord, most commonly in the territory of the artery of Adamkiewicz. In this case, ischaemia predominantly affects the anterior two-thirds of the spinal cord, while sparing the posterior columns.

The most frequent site of spinal cord infarction is the thoracolumbar junction.

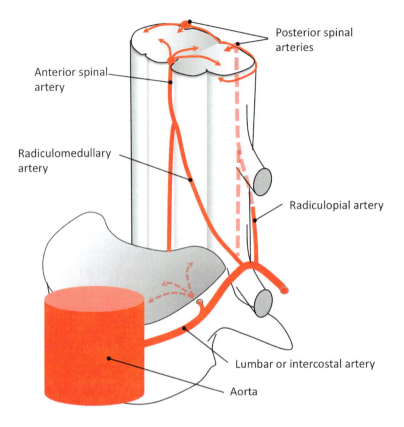

Fig. 11.1 Arterial vascular anatomy of the spinal cord

Clinical Features

- Spinal cord infarction is very rare compared to cerebral infarction due to the small dimensions of the spinal cord, the abundance of arterial anastomoses and the low incidence of atherosclerosis of spinal arteries.
- Clinical symptoms are very variable, depending on the level and depth of ischaemia.
- Neurological disorders with sudden or very rapidly progressive onset, often preceded by back pain. Very rarely, some patients report previous episodes of transient neurological deficits (spinal cord TIA).
- Most classical clinical presentation: anterior spinal syndrome characterized by sudden onset of painful paraparesis or tetraparesis with sensory deficit for pain and temperature below the lesion, sphincter disorders and relative sparing of deep sensation. The level of the lesion is usually cervicothoracic or thoraco-lumbar (due to the anatomical arrangement of the blood supply). Differential

diagnosis with transverse myelitis can sometimes be difficult. Imaging is useful to differentiate between the two entities. Possibility of incomplete Brown-Séquard syndrome (hemiparesis ipsilateral to the lesion and contralateral pain and temperature sensory deficit with sparing of deep sensation in this context) in case of unilateral involvement.

- Posterior spinal syndrome is much rarer due to the extensive anastomotic networks. Generally bilateral involvement, responsible for paraesthesia and disorders of deep sensation, sometimes with motor and spinothalamic involvement in the case of anterior extension. If unilateral involvement (rare), incomplete Brown-Séquard syndrome with sparing of pain and temperature sensitivity.

Aetiologies

- Iatrogenic: aortic surgery, thoracic surgery, arteriography, epidural anaesthesia, spinal anaesthesia and foraminal steroid infiltration.
- Spontaneous: vertebral artery occlusion (cervical spinal cord infarction), aortic diseases (thoracolumbar spinal cord infarction), aortic or vertebral artery atherosclerosis and dissection, emboligenic heart disease.
- Rare: fibrocartilaginous embolism. Young patients, mainly women, after physical exercise. Mechanism: embolus from disk material.

Investigations

CT aortography looking for atherosclerosis, dissection and coarctation. Carotid Doppler and transcranial Doppler looking for vertebral artery occlusion in the case of superior cervical or thoracic spinal cord infarction.

TTE ± TOE looking for cardiac causes.

Imaging

CT

Often normal. Sometimes vertebral bone infarct (detected on follow-up imaging).

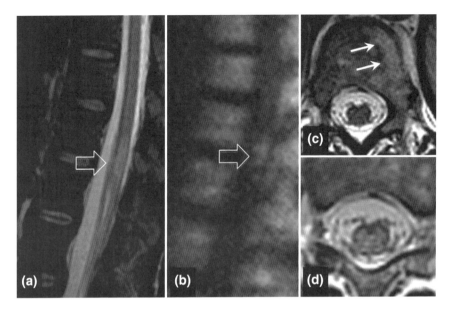

Fig. 11.2 Spinal cord infarction of the conus medullaris. Sagittal section on MRI T2-weighted images (**a**) shows the hyperintense conus medullaris infarction (*hollow arrow*), confirmed by axial section (**d**). The diffusion-weighted sequence also shows hyperintensity of the conus medullaris (**b** *hollow arrow*) corresponding to the abnormalities visible on T2-weighted images. Association of an overlying hyperintense vertebral bone infarction in the left part of the vertebral body (**c** *double arrows*). Note the normal signal of the spinal cord at this level (**c**) compared to the infarcted spinal cord segment (**d**)

MRI (Figs. 11.2 and 11.3)

Centromedullary hyperintensity on T2-weighted images if anterior spinal artery, or posterior peripheral hyperintensity if posterior spinal artery. Hyperintense signal on diffusion-weighted images with low ADC. Hemivertebral infarction with hyperintense signal on T2-weighted images (T2-weighted inversion-recovery sequences ++).

Outcome

- Prognosis often very poor. 20 % mortality at the acute phase (especially cervical spinal cord infarction). Disabling sequelae in 50–60 % of patients, particularly after infarction of the anterior spinal artery territory: paraplegia, persistent sphincter disorders.
- Good prognosis in the absence of proprioceptive and sphincter disorders, and incomplete paraplegia at the acute phase.

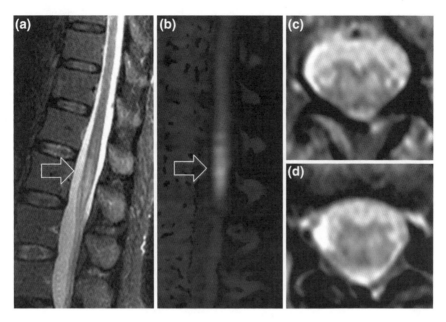

Fig. 11.3 Spinal cord infarction of the conus medullaris. Sagittal section on MRI T2-weighted images (**a**) shows the hyperintense conus medullaris infarction (*hollow arrow*), confirmed by axial section (**c** and **d**). The diffusion-weighted sequence also shows hyperintensity of the conus medullaris (**b** *hollow arrow*) corresponding to the abnormalities visible on T2-weighted images

Treatment

No drug therapy has been evaluated. In practice, initiation of antiplatelet therapy, prevention of bedsore complications, and rehabilitation.

Selected References

1. Thurnher MM, Bammer R (2006) Diffusion-weighted MR imaging (DWI) in spinal cord ischemia. Neuroradiology 48:795–801
2. Nedeltchev K et al (2004) Long-term outcome of acute spinal cord ischemia syndrome. Stroke 35:560–565
3. Brochier T, Ceccaldi M, Milandre L, Brouchon M (1999) Dorsolateral infarction of the lower medulla: clinical-MRI study. Neurology 1(52)190–193
4. Faig J et al (1998) Vertebral body infarction as a confirmatory sign of spinal cord ischemic stroke: report of three cases and review of the literature. Stroke 29:239–243
5. Masson C et al (2004) Spinal cord infarction: clinical and MRI findings and short-term outcome. J Neurol Neurosurg Psychiatry 75:1431–1435

Chapter 12
Radiological Differential Diagnosis of Cerebral Infarction

Leukoaraiosis

Definition

The term '*Leukoaraiosis*' means rarefaction of the white matter. It is a radiological definition and not a histological definition. Leukoaraiosis results from chronic ischaemia due to diseases of small perforating arteries supplying the white matter.

Clinical Features

Leukoaraiosis is a nonspecific sign that becomes more extensive with age. It is often associated with lacunar infarcts, dilated Virchow-Robin spaces and microbleeds. Leukoaraiosis is observed more frequently in patients with vascular dementia, cerebral infarction and cerebral haemorrhage than in healthy subjects.

Imaging

Focal and confluent hypodensities (CT) or hyperintensities on T2-weighted and FLAIR images (MRI) of the periventricular and subcortical white matter. According to Brant-Zawadzki's classification, four grades are defined depending on the extent of visible abnormalities (Fig. 12.1).

Multiple Sclerosis (Fig. 12.2)

Inflammatory disease of the central nervous system characterized by demyelinating lesions of the white matter affecting young subjects (age of onset generally between 20 and 40 years), mainly women. The first episode of multiple sclerosis

G. Saliou et al., *Practical Guide to Neurovascular Emergencies*,
DOI: 10.1007/978-2-8178-0481-1_12, © Springer-Verlag France 2014

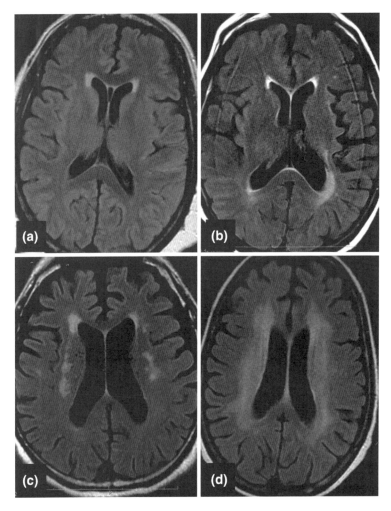

Fig. 12.1 Four grades of leukoaraiosis according to Brant-Zawadzki's classification in 4 different patients. Grade 1 **a** occasional frontal periventricular hyperintensities. Grade 2 **b** hyperintensities visible in the occipital horns. Grade 3 **c** diffuse periventricular nonconfluent hyperintensities. Grade 4 **d** confluent and diffuse periventricular white matter hyperintensities

(MS) can sometimes be mistaken for an infarct, as it can sometimes have a sudden onset (symptoms generally progress over several days or sometimes several hours).

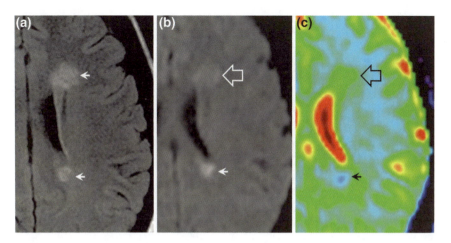

Fig. 12.2 Multiple sclerosis on MRI. Two lesions appear hyperintense on FLAIR images (**a** *arrows*). On diffusion-weighted images, they have different appearances: one lesion is hyperintense (**b** *arrow*) with decreased ADC (**c** *arrow*) and the other lesion is isointense (**b** *hollow arrow*) with an increased ADC (**c** *hollow arrow*)

Imaging

MRI

No grey matter lesions (cortex and basal ganglia). Isolated white matter lesion, predominantly supratentorial. Old lesions present a normal or increased ADC, while recent (active) lesions can present a decreased ADC. Oval-shaped (rather than rounded) hyperintensities, often multiple, with a long axis perpendicular to the ventricles are observed on T2-weighted and FLAIR images.

Frequent involvement of the corpus callosum and cervical spine (cervical MRI should be performed when in doubt). Possible contrast enhancement of recent plaques.

Tumours

Progressive onset of neurological deficit. Symptoms of intracranial hypertension are frequently present. The neurological deficit can appear suddenly in the case of intratumoural bleeding. The most common tumours are brain metastases (Fig. 12.3), gliomas and lymphomas (Fig. 12.4).

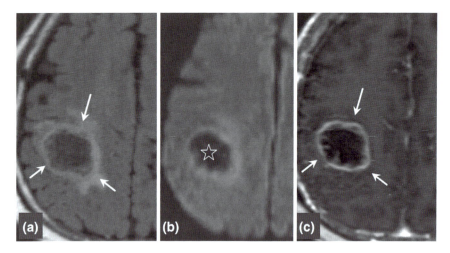

Fig. 12.3 Brain metastasis on MRI. The lesion has a heterogeneous appearance on FLAIR images with a hyperintense margin (**a** *arrows*) and a hypointense centre. On diffusion-weighted imaging, the lesion is hypointense (**b**) associated with an increased ADC. On the gadolinium-enhanced sequence, contrast enhancement of the tumour wall (**c** *arrows*) with no enhancement of the necrotic centre

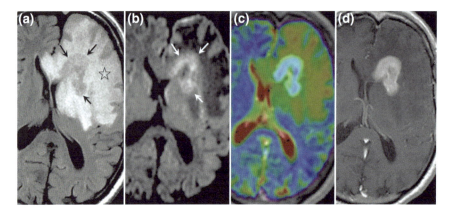

Fig. 12.4 Primary lymphoma of the brain. The lesion is hyperintense on FLAIR images (**a** *arrows*), with extensive perilesional oedema (**a** *star*), hyperintense on diffusion-weighted images (**b** *arrows*) with decreased ADC (**c** ADC map; the lesion is blue due to decreased ADC). Gadolinium enhancement of the lesion (**d**)

Imaging

Mass effect on adjacent structures. No systematized vascular territory involvement. Contrast enhancement may be observed. Necrotic zones present an increased ADC (hypointense on diffusion-weighted images). Note that tumours can bleed (particularly metastases) and may initially be mistaken for haematoma.

Infections

Abscess (Fig. 12.5)

- Clinical setting of sepsis and sometimes immunodepression.
- Note that fever is often absent.
- Usually rapidly progressive deficit.

Imaging

A marked mass effect on adjacent structures and hyperintense perilesional oedema are generally observed on T2-weighted and FLAIR images. Hyperintensity on diffusion-weighted images (decreased ADC) or normal diffusion. Annular contrast enhancement of the wall. No systematized arterial involvement.

Encephalitis (Figs. 12.6 and 12.7)

- Specific features depending on the cause (infectious, metabolic, toxic, etc.).
- Rapidly progressive, rather than sudden onset of disorders.
- Disorders of consciousness (obtundation, confusion, coma) are almost constantly present.
- Seizures are frequently associated.

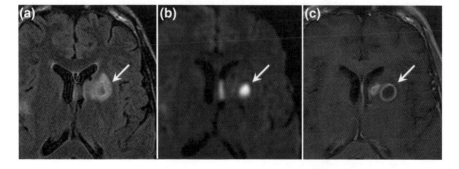

Fig. 12.5 Pyogenic brain abscess on MRI. The lesion is hyperintense on FLAIR images (**a** *arrow*) with a less intense centre. On diffusion-weighted images (**b** *arrow*), the lesion is hyperintense (limited diffusion with decreased ADC) Gadolinium enhancement of the abscess wall (**c** *arrow*)

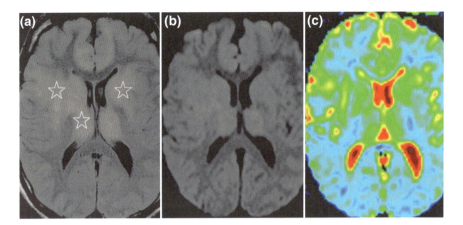

Fig. 12.6 MRI of infectious encephalitis in a patient with AIDS, involving the frontal lobes and basal ganglia. On FLAIR images, the lesions are hyperintense (**a** *stars*), disseminated and do not correspond to an arterial territory. On diffusion-weighted images, the lesions are isointense (**b**) due to moderately increased ADC caused by vasogenic oedema (**c**)

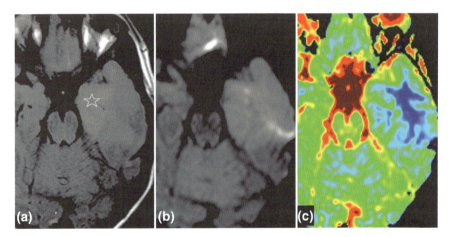

Fig. 12.7 Herpetic encephalitis involving the temporal lobes, predominantly on the left side. On FLAIR images, the lesions are hyperintense (**a** *star*), disseminated and do not correspond to an arterial territory. On diffusion-weighted images, the lesions are hyperintense (**b**) due to moderately decreased ADC caused by cytotoxic oedema (**c**)

Imaging

Parenchymal oedema (hyperintensity on FLAIR and T2-weighted images, hypo-density on CT) with moderate mass effect on adjacent structures. Normal or elevated ADC due to vasogenic oedema (iso- or hypointense on diffusion-weighted images), sometimes decreased (hyperintense on diffusion-weighted images). ADC is markedly decreased in the presence of abscess.

Disruption of blood–brain barrier with possible contrast enhancement of parenchyma. On perfusion-weighted images: prolonged MTT due to oedema; CBV is maintained or only moderately decreased

PRES (Posterior Reversible Encephalopathy Syndrome) (Fig. 12.8)

Definition

PRES is a radiological syndrome and not a clinical syndrome. Vasogenic oedema due to disruption of the arteriolar blood–brain barrier. The abnormalities are reversible. Haemorrhage may be associated in 15 % of cases (meningeal haemorrhage, cerebral haemorrhage or microbleeds), independently of blood pressure, depending on the aetiology.

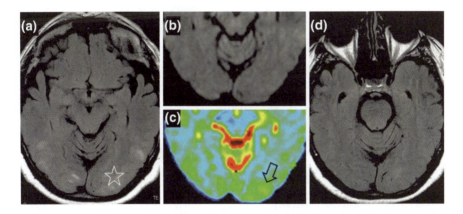

Fig. 12.8 Hypertensive encephalopathy in a patient with headache associated with bilateral blindness in a context of hypertensive crisis. FLAIR sequence at the acute phase shows multiple cortical/subcortical hyperintensities clearly predominant in the occipital regions (**a** *star*). Diffusion-weighted images (**b**) and ADC colour mapping show typical vasogenic cerebral oedema with increased ADC (**c** *hollow arrow*) and isointense signal on diffusion-weighted images compared to healthy cerebral parenchyma. The follow-up FLAIR sequence (**d**) demonstrates the reversible nature of the lesions after correction of blood pressure, with resolution of the initial hyperintensities

Clinical Features

Most common symptoms: headache, seizures, confusion. Can occur at any age.

Multiple Aetiologies

Acute or subacute HT is the leading cause, eclampsia, autoimmune diseases, immunosuppression (organ transplantation, allogeneic bone marrow transplantation), reversible cerebral vasoconstriction syndrome, sepsis, chemotherapy. When PRES is due to allogeneic transplantation or sepsis, it is associated with haemorrhage in 33 % of cases!

IMAGING

CT

Bilateral cortical and subcortical hypodensities predominantly in the occipital region. The brainstem or basal ganglia are more rarely involved

Possible iodinated contrast enhancement (disruption of the blood–brain barrier).Hyperdensity indicating haemorrhage must be systematically investigated.

MRI

Bilateral cortical and subcortical hyperintensities on T2-weighted and FLAIR sequences with posterior occipital predominance. Possible involvement of basal ganglia. ADC increased or normal (hypointensity or normal on diffusion-weighted images) related to vasogenic oedema.

Possible gadolinium enhancement. Cortical sulci are hyperintense on FLAIR images and hypointense on T2*-weighted images in the case of meningeal haemorrhage. Focal intraparenchymal hypointensity on T2*-weighted images in the case of microbleed. Variable signal depending on the age of the haematoma.

Treatment

Blood pressure control. Treatment of the cause whenever possible (extraction of foetus in the case of eclampsia).

Metabolic Infarction

Melas (Fig. 12.9)

Definition

MELAS = *Mitochondrial Encephalopathy, Lactic Acidosis and Stroke-like episodes*. Maternally inherited genetic disorder affecting children and young adults (mean age of onset of symptoms around 15 years), with headache, seizures, and predominantly occipital lobe infarction. Zones of old and recent ischaemia are observed on imaging, not corresponding to the usual arterial territories.

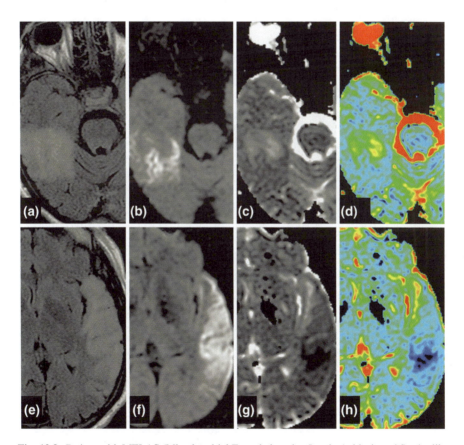

Fig. 12.9 Patient with MELAS (Mitochondrial Encephalopathy, Lactic Acidosis and Stroke-like episodes). Infarcts of various ages. Old right temporal infarct (**a** axial FLAIR). Hyperintensity on diffusion-weighted imaging (**b** diffusion) related to the T2 effect, as ADC is increased, and hyperintensity on ADC mapping (**c**). Perfusion is normal (**d** cerebral blood volume mapping). In contrast, recent left parietotemporal infarction (**e** axial FLAIR sequence), hyperintensity on diffusion-weighted imaging (**f**) with decreased ADC and hypointensity (**g**) and restriction on perfusion-weighted imaging (**h** increased CBV shown in *blue*)

Imaging

CT

Recent, hypodense focal infarction not corresponding to a specific arterial territory, associated with ischaemic sequelae visualized as more marked lacunar hypodensities or cerebral atrophy.

MRI

Zones cortical or cortical/subcortical infarction of various ages, not corresponding to a specific arterial territory, with hyperintensity on T2-weighted and FLAIR images and variable signal on diffusion-weighted images depending on the age of the infarct. Characteristic lactate peaks at 1.3 ppm on spectroscopy in approximately two-thirds of patients in normal brain parenchyma remote to the abnormalities.

Seizures (Fig. 12.10)

Clinical Features

Generalized Seizure

Loss of consciousness (rare in infarction). Postictal confusion with prolonged anterograde amnesia. Clinical history must look for tonic–clonic movements, tongue biting and incontinence. Possible post-critical deficit, particularly in the case of secondarily generalized seizures, followed by complete recovery, which may take several days, especially in the presence of an underlying lesion (Todd's paralysis).

Partial Seizure

Very brief neurological deficit (maximum 5 min). Possible myoclonic seizures. A more prolonged deficit may be observed after partial status epilepticus (need for EEG).

A first seizure is rare (5 %) in the context of ischaemic stroke (more frequent in the case of cardioembolic stroke), and more frequent in the context of haemorrhagic stroke (cortical haematoma).

Pathophysiology

Cerebral ischaemia is a rare complication of seizures and can occur in a context of status epilepticus lasting more than 30 min. An initial phase of compensation of

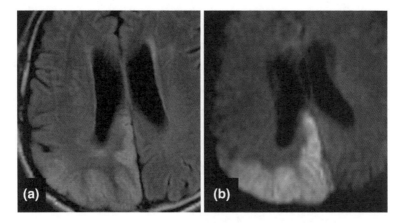

Fig. 12.10 Patient with status epilepticus. Parietal cortical abnormalities (**a** FLAIR image, **b** diffusion-weighted image), not corresponding to an arterial territory, but located in the seizure focus. Cytotoxic oedema is due to onset of anaerobic metabolism due to excessive local glucose consumption associated with neuronal hyperactivation. These abnormalities are reversible

metabolic needs may be followed by a second decompensation phase. Neuronal ischaemia is therefore related to excessive intracellular glucose consumption during the seizure, leading to loss of cerebral autoregulation with hypoxia and elevation of lactic acid levels, resulting in cytotoxic and/or vasogenic oedema, possibly leading to neuronal cell death.

Imaging

Imaging can be normal. Vasogenic or cytotoxic oedema can affect most regions of the brain: cortex, white matter, meninges, corpus callosum and hippocampus. The zone of oedema does not correspond to an arterial territory. The abnormalities resolve after treatment of the seizure. In case of prolonged seizures, cytotoxic oedema can lead to irreversible lesions on imaging.

CT

Focal or more extensive hypodensity associated with a possible mass effect on adjacent structures (effacement of cortical sulci).

MRI

Hyperintensity on T2-weighted and FLAIR images with decreased ADC (hyper-intense on diffusion-weighted images) in the presence of cytotoxic oedema and/or increased ADC (hypointense on diffusion-weighted images) in the presence of vasogenic oedema. Possible cortical or leptomeningeal gadolinium enhancement due to disruption of the blood–brain barrier.

Transient Lesion in the Splenium of the Corpus Callosum (Fig. 12.11)

The presence of localized MRI abnormalities in the splenium of the corpus callosum is classically observed in a number of metabolic disorders. After correction of these metabolic abnormalities, the MRI abnormalities can also be reversible. The mechanisms involved are focal oedema (vasogenic and/or cytotoxic) or focal demyelination.

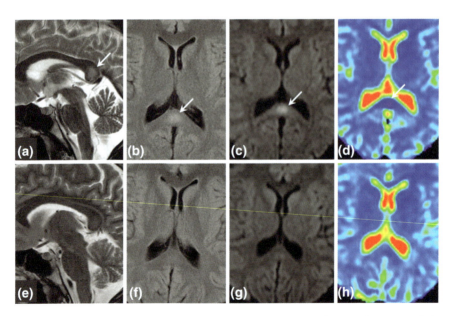

Fig. 12.11 Hyperintensity on T2-weighted (**a** *arrow*) and FLAIR images (**b** *arrow*) of the splenium of the corpus callosum associated with hypoglycaemia. Hyperintense appearance on diffusion-weighted images (**c** *arrow*) with decreased ADC (**d** *arrow*). Marked regression of the abnormalities on follow-up MRI (**e, f, g** and **h**) on D10 after correction of blood glucose

Clinical Features

Clinical features are nonspecific and variable: confusion, ataxia, epilepsy, dysarthria, hemispheric disconnection (left-sided ideomotor apraxia, left-sided tactile anomia, constructive apraxia of the right hand).

Aetiologies

Alcoholism, malnutrition, encephalitis (HSV, HIV, Rotavirus, Salmonella, *E. coli*, malaria), ADEM (acute disseminated encephalomyelitis), epilepsy, drug therapy (antiepileptic drugs, chemotherapy), hypoglycaemia, hypo- and hypernatraemia, ischaemic stroke, HT, renal failure.

Imaging

CT

Focal hypodensity of the splenium of the corpus callosum.

MRI

Hyperintensity on T2-weighted and FLAIR images in the splenium of the corpus callosum. Cytotoxic oedema with restricted diffusion and decreased ADC. Possible gadolinium enhancement.

Migraine

Migraine with aura can be a differential diagnosis of TIA.

Imaging

MRI

Small hyperintensities of the deep white matter (Fig. 12.12) and small cerebellar infarcts (Fig. 12.13) are observed more frequently than in nonmigrainous subjects in the case of frequent attacks of migraine with aura. Unknown significance.

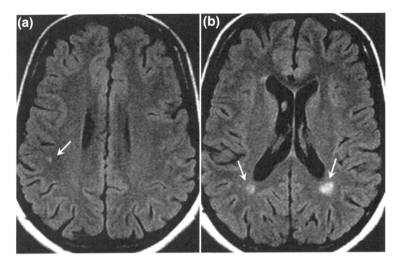

Fig. 12.12 21-year-old female patient with frequent migraines with aura. MRI FLAIR sequence discloses nonspecific subcortical (**a** *arrow*) and periventricular (**b** *arrows*) white matter hyperintensities

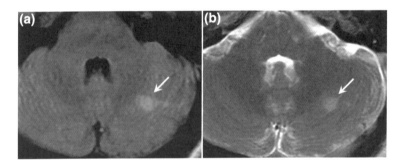

Fig. 12.13 47-year-old female patient with frequent migraines with aura. MRI FLAIR sequence (**a**) and T2-weighted SE image (**b**) shows a hyperintense focal left cerebellar infarct scar (*arrows*). This type of abnormality is observed more frequently in migrainous patients

Normal MRI in familial hemiplegic migraine. N.B.: migraine with aura may be a symptom of various brain disorders (arteriovenous malformation, CADASIL, etc.).

Selected References

1. Brant-Zawadzki M et al (1985) MR. Imaging of the aging brain: patchy white-matter lesions and dementia. AJNR 6:675–682
2. Hachinski VC et al (1987) Leuko-araiosis. Arch Neurol 44:21–23
3. Hinchey J et al (1996) A reversible posterior leukoencephalopathy syndrome. N Engl J Med 334:494–500

4. Casey SO et al (2000) Posterior reversible encephalopathy syndrome: utility of fluid-attenuated inversion recovery MR imaging in the detection of cortical and subcortical lesions. AJNR 21:1199–1206

5. Provenzale JM et al (2001) Quantitative assessment of diffusion abnormalities in posterior réversible encephalopathy syndrome. AJNR 22:1455–1461

6. Schwartz R et al (2009) Catheter angiography, MR angiography, and MR perfusion in posterior reversible encephalopathy syndrome. AJNR 30:E19

7. Hefzy HM et al (2009) Hemorrhage in posterior reversible encephalopathy syndrome: imaging and clinical features. AJNR 30:1371–1379

8. Pavlakis SG et al (1984) Mitochondrial myopathy, encephalopathy, lactic acidosis, and strokelike episodes: a distinctive clinical syndrome. Ann Neurol 16:481–488

9. Allard JC et al (1988) CT and MR of MELAS syndrome. AJNR Am J Neuroradiol 9:1234–1238

10. Abe K (2004) Comparison of conventional and diffusion-weighted MRI and proton MR spectroscopy in patients with mitochondrial encephalomyopathy, lactic acidosis, and stroke-like events. Neuroradiology 46:113–117

11. Ong B et al (2009) Transient seizure-related MRI abnormalities. J Neuroimaging 19:301–310

12. Nair PP et al (2009) Role of cranial imaging in epileptic status. Eur J Radiol 70:475–480

13. Kim JA et al (2001) Transient MR signal changes in patients with generalized tonicoclonic seizure or status epilepticus: preictal diffusion-weighted imaging. AJNR 22:1149–1160

14. Da Rocha AJ et al (2006) Focal transient lesion in the splenium of the corpus callosum in three non-epileptic patients. Neuroradiology 48:731–735

15. Doherty MJ et al (2005) Clinical implications of splenium magnetic resonance imaging signal changes. Arch Neurol 62:433–437

16. Kruit MC et al (2004) Migraine as a risk factor for subclinical brain lesions. JAMA 28(291)427–434

Chapter 13
Incidental Findings

Nonspecific White Matter Changes (Hyperintensities)

Definition

A few scattered white matter hyperintensities on FLAIR and T2-weighted images, not corresponding to demyelinating, vascular, metabolic or toxic diseases.

Clinical Features

Incidental finding. Prevalence on MRI: <1 % before the age of 30, 3 % between the ages of 30 and 50, 7 % between the ages of 50 and 70 and 18 % between the ages of 70 and 90. No associated with any clinical features. Increase in number and size with age and blood pressure. More frequent in the case of migraine with aura, smoking, atrial fibrillation and atherosclerosis.

Associated with an increased risk of cognitive impairment, stroke and decreased life expectancy.

Aetiology

Undetermined. Resembles leukoaraiosis.

Imaging

Can be detected on MRI T2-weighted and FLAIR sequences (Fig. 13.1), but not visible or only poorly visible on other sequences. Variable numbers of isolated, scattered, small hypersignals, without contrast enhancement or mass effect.

G. Saliou et al., *Practical Guide to Neurovascular Emergencies*,
DOI: 10.1007/978-2-8178-0481-1_13, © Springer-Verlag France 2014

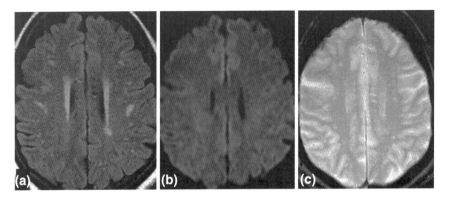

Fig. 13.1 Incidental finding on MRI (**a** FLAIR sequence) of numerous focal white matter hyperintensities in a 54-year-old female patient with no particular history investigated for nonspecific chronic headache. The patient was otherwise asymptomatic. Note the absence of any abnormality suggestive of recent ischaemic or haemorrhagic lesion on the other sequences (**b** diffusion-weighted images, **c** T2*-weighted images)

Ubiquitous topography but preferentially located at the cortical-subcortical junction. Lesions become stable with time. No associated spinal cord abnormalities on MRI.

Management

No specific monitoring in the absence of symptoms.

Unruptured Aneurysm (Fig. 13.2)

Prevalence of 2–5 % in the general population.

An intracranial aneurysm is a frequent incidental finding on imaging (MRI, CT angiography) and is the second most common incidental finding after silent infarcts on brain MRI procedure, detected on 0.23–1.8 % of MRI examinations.

Size at the time of discovery often <7 mm and often in the carotid territory.

Imaging

CT

Spontaneously isodense. Sometimes fine mural calcifications. Intensive contrast enhancement.

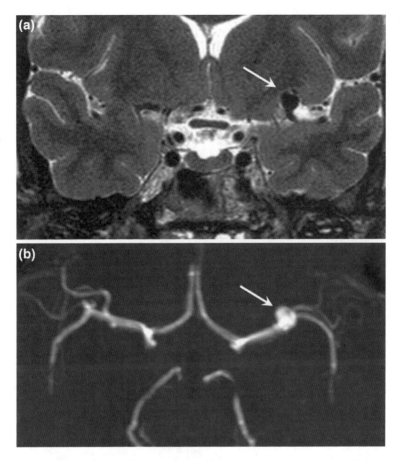

Fig. 13.2 Incidental finding of unruptured intracranial aneurysm on brain MRI in a young female patient. The aneurysm is hypointense on the T2-weighted SE image (**a** *arrow*, coronal section). The TOF sequence (**b** *arrow*, axial reconstruction) confirms the presence of the saccular aneurysm at the left middle cerebral artery bifurcation

MRI

Additional image on TOF sequence, clearly visible as hypointensity on T2-weighted SE images.

Pulse artifact around the aneurysm. Early intensive gadolinium enhancement.

A large aneurysm can cause a mass effect on adjacent structures with hyperintense perianeurysmal oedema on T2-weighted and FLAIR images.

Management

No randomized study has been conducted.

Consultation with an interventional neuroradiologist or neurosurgeon to determine the management strategy: simple surveillance or endovascular or surgical treatment according to criteria associated with an increased risk of spontaneous rupture of the aneurysm.

The two main factors associated with an increased risk of rupture are the size of the aneurysm >7 mm and smoking. Other factors are also known to increase the risk of rupture: alcoholism, hypertension, family history of ruptured intracranial aneurysm and vertebrobasilar or posterior communicating artery aneurysms.

Developmental Venous Anomaly (Fig. 13.3)

Developmental venous anomalies are also called venous angiomas.

The superficial cerebral venous drainage is ensured by superficial cortical veins. The deep venous drainage is ensured by deep cerebral veins. The superficial and deep venous networks communicate via transcortical veins that are not visible or only barely visible on imaging.

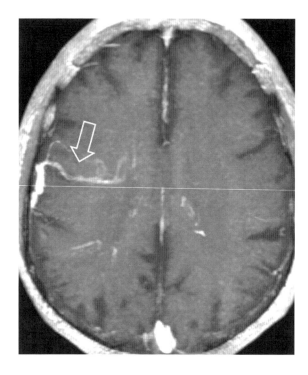

Fig. 13.3 Gadolinium-enhanced MRI T1-weighted sequence showing a superficial developmental venous anomaly draining the deep part of the brain (*hollow arrow*). The transcortical vein drains into an enlarged normal cortical vein related to a larger draining territory compared with other cortical veins

Developmental venous anomaly: superficial venous drainage of a deep territory or deep venous drainage of a superficial territory via a dilated transcortical vein located in a cerebral hemisphere or the cerebellum, but never in the brainstem or spinal cord.

Frequently associated with cerebral cavernous malformation, or more rarely with arteriovenous malformation, sinus pericranii, anomaly of cortical gyri (pachygyria, schizo-encephalopathy), venous or sinus ectasia, capillary telangiectasia.

Clinical Features

Asymptomatic when the anomaly is isolated.

Like any cerebral vein, a DVA can become thrombosed. In the case of thrombosis: investigations and treatment identical to classical cerebral venous thromboses after eliminating an underlying ruptured arteriovenous malformation by arteriography.

Imaging

Typical "jellyfish head" or umbrella appearance on gadolinium-enhanced MRI T1-weighted volume-rendering sequence or contrast-enhanced CT scan. On perfusion-weighted images, normal MTT, CBV increased sometimes due to increased local venous blood volume. Normal diffusion-weighted images.

Capillary Telangiectasia (Fig. 13.4)

Asymptomatic focal capillary dilatation in normal cerebral parenchyma, generally isolated and an incidental finding. Can occur anywhere in the brain, but frequent in the brainstem. May develop after radiotherapy. Sometimes associated with a developmental venous anomaly or, more rarely, with Osler-Weber-Rendu disease, especially when associated with cerebral arteriovenous malformations (micro-AVM or pial fistulas).

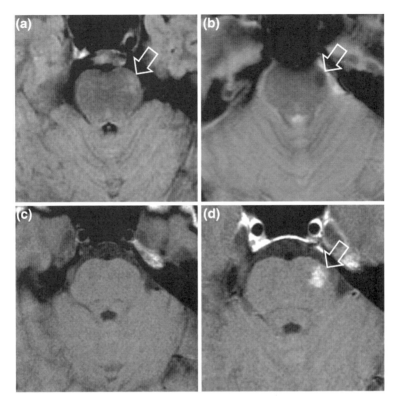

Fig. 13.4 Telangiectasia of brainstem on MRI. The characteristic appearance is moderately hyperintense on FLAIR (**a** *hollow arrow*) and T2-weighted SE images and moderately hypointense on T2-weighted GE images (**b** *hollow arrow*). The anomaly is not visible on T1-weighted images (**c**) and shows homogeneous gadolinium enhancement (**d** *hollow arrow*)

Imaging

CT

Normal. Focal zone of iodinated contrast enhancement.

MRI

Fairly characteristic hypointense appearance on T2*-weighted images and not visible or moderately hyperintense on FLAIR and T2-weighted SE images. Not visible on T1-weighted images. No mass effect on adjacent structures. Homogeneous gadolinium enhancement.

Management

No treatment is required for isolated telangiectasia. Benign incidental finding. Exclude Osler-Weber-Rendu disease in young subjects and an associated true AVM.

Fibromuscular Dysplasia (Fig. 13.5)

This non-atheromatous, non-inflammatory disease of uncertain origin involves medium-sized muscular arteries, mainly renal arteries (60 % of cases) and extracranial carotid arteries (30 % of cases). It consists of a succession of stenoses and dilatations with a "string of pearls" appearance. Stenoses are due to three

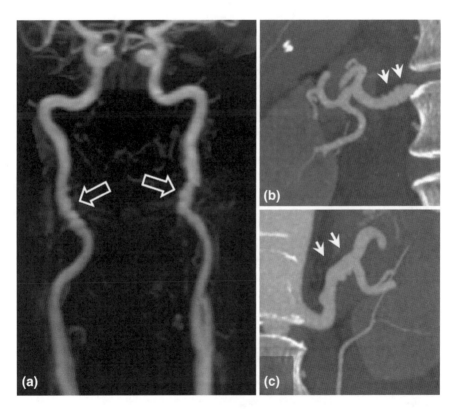

Fig. 13.5 Fibromuscular dysplasia in a 68-year-old female patient. Note the characteristic "pile of plates" appearance of successive internal carotid artery stenoses (**a** cerebral MR angiography, *hollow arrows*). CT angiography of renal arteries also reveals a suggestive moniliform appearance (**b** and **c** *double arrows*). *By courtesy of Dr. Olivier Naggara, hôpital Sainte-Anne, Paris*

types of fibrous hyperplasia : medial (60–70 %, involvement of internal elastic lamina), perimedial or subadventitial (10–20 %, involvement of outer layer of the media) or intimal (5 %, involvement of the intima).

In 11 % of cases, familial form with characteristic appearance on imaging in at least one relative.

Clinical Features

Generally asymptomatic. Link with an increased risk of cerebral infarction has not been proven. Risk factor for arterial dissection (20 % of carotid artery dissections are associated with renal or cervical FMD), arteriovenous fistula and intracranial aneurysm.

Imaging

CT Angiography, MR Angiography of Head and Neck and Arteriography

Succession of internal carotid artery stenoses with typical "pile of plates" or "string of pearls" (moniliform) appearance.

External carotid and vertebrobasilar arteries not affected.

Treatment

No specific treatment recommended if asymptomatic.

If detected after cerebral infarction, aspirin is recommended as secondary prevention but with no evidence of its efficacy.

If tight stenosis with haemodynamic consequences, surgical or endovascular treatment (angioplasty ± stenting) should be considered.

Selected References

1. Ylikoski A et al (1995) White matter hyperintensities on MRI in the neurologically nondiseased elderly. Analysis of cohorts of consecutive subjects aged 55 to 85 years living at home. Stroke 26:1171–1177
2. Kuller LH et al (2004) Cardiovascular health study collaborative research group. White matter hyperintensity on cranial magnetic resonance imaging: a predictor of stroke. Stroke 35:1821–1825

3. Morris Z et al (2009) Incidental findings on brain magnetic resonance imaging: systematic review and meta-analysis. BMJ 17(339):b3016
4. Vernooij MW et al (2007) Incidental findings on brain MRI in the general population. N Engl J Med 1(357)1821–1828
5. Molyneux A et al (2002) International subarachnoid aneurysm trial (ISAT) collaborative group. International subarachnoid aneurysm trial (ISAT) of neurosurgical clipping versus endovascular coiling in 2143 patients with ruptured intracranial aneurysms: a randomised trial. Lancet 26(360)1267–1274
6. Wiebers DO et al (2003) International study of unruptured intracranial aneurysms investigators. Unruptured intracranial aneurysms: natural history, clinical outcome, and risks of surgical and endovascular treatment. Lancet12(362)103–110
7. Jimenez JL et al (1989) The trans-cerebral veins: normal and non-pathologic angiographic aspects. Surg Radiol Anat 11:63–72
8. Goulao A et al (1990) Venous anomalies and abnormalities of the posterior fossa. Neuroradiology 31:476–482
9. Leary MC et al (2004) Cerebrovascular complications of fibromuscular dysplasia. Curr Treat Options Cardiovasc Med 6:237–248
10. So EL et al (1981) Cephalic fibromuscular dysplasia in 32 patients: clinical findings and radiologic features. Arch Neurol 38:619–622

Chapter 14
Thrombolysis

Intravenous Thrombolysis

Objectives

To dissolve (lyse) a thrombus obstructing an artery in order to restore perfusion pressure.

Most effective single treatment of cerebral infarction, especially when it is performed at an early stage. Currently only performed in less than 13 % of patients.

Allows complete recanalisation in almost 50 % of cases of middle cerebral artery occlusion (Fig. 14.1), but a much lower rate in the case of carotid artery occlusion.

Increases the chances of recovery without sequelae or with only minor sequelae by 30 %.

Allows recovery of one in eight patients (Fig. 14.2), despite an increased incidence of symptomatic cerebral haemorrhage (6.4 % *versus* 0.6 % with placebo), without significantly altering the mortality.

Indications

Intravenous thrombolysis should be considered for all cases of suspected infarction with onset of symptoms within the last 4.5 h. Treatment must not be administered if time of onset of symptoms cannot be determined with certainty (for example, presence of a deficit upon waking in the morning).

Strokes in diffusion-weighted images with unknown onset could be consider for thrombolysis if FLAIR sequence is normal, which means that stroke onset is probably less than 3 h (off-label indication).

G. Saliou et al., *Practical Guide to Neurovascular Emergencies*,
DOI: 10.1007/978-2-8178-0481-1_14, © Springer-Verlag France 2014

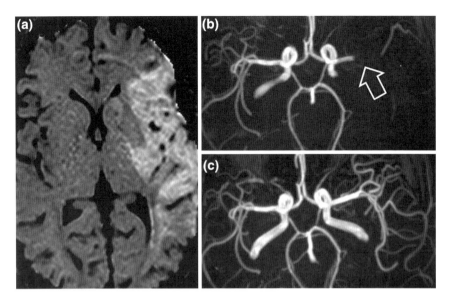

Fig. 14.1 22-year-old female patient with left middle cerebral artery infarction and right hemiplegia and aphasia. The NIHSS score was 20. MRI performed 3 h after onset of symptoms shows abnormalities on diffusion-weighted images in the left superficial middle cerebral artery territory (**a** diffusion-weighted sequence) with occlusion of the left middle cerebral artery bifurcation (**b** TOF sequence, *hollow arrow*). Resolution of the arterial occlusion after intravenous thrombolysis on follow-up MRI (**c** TOF sequence) with improvement of the neurological state and recovery of hemiplegia (NIHSS = 6)

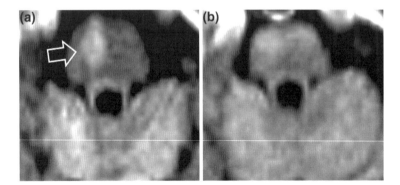

Fig. 14.2 78-year-old female patient with a right paramedian bulbar infarct with left hemiplegia. The NIHSS score was 12. MRI performed 1.5 h after the onset of symptoms shows a slightly decreased ADC with moderately hyperintense signal in the medulla oblongata (**a** diffusion-weighted sequence, *hollow arrow*). Fifteen minutes after the start of intravenous thrombolysis, complete recovery of all neurological symptoms (NIHSS = 0). Normal diffusion-weighted images on 24-hour follow-up MRI (**b**)

Contraindications

(as defined in the SPC for Actilyse®)

Main risk factor for post-thrombolysis fatal cerebral haemorrhage is failure to comply with contraindications:

- History:

    - cerebral infarction, severe head injury within the last three months;
    - diabetic patient with a history of stroke;
    - cerebral haemorrhage;
    - gastrointestinal or urinary tract haemorrhage within the last 21 days;
    - recent myocardial infarction;
    - recent puncture of a non-compressible vessel;
    - intercurrent disease;
    - bacterial endocarditis, pericarditis, pancreatitis, severe liver disease.

- Clinical features:

    - SBP > 185 and/or DBP > 110 at the time of administration of the product;
    - minor or rapidly resolving neurological deficit, such as an isolated sensory deficit, isolated ataxia, isolated dysarthria or minor motor deficit (in practice when NIHSS < 5 [refer to Appendix 1]);
    - severe neurological deficit (NIHSS > 22), deep coma;
    - seizures at the time of onset of the disorders (relative IC).

- Laboratory parameters:

    - Ongoing anticoagulant treatment or INR > 1.7;
    - Heparin within the last 24 h and prolonged APTT;
    - Platelet count <100,000/mm^3;
    - Blood glucose <0.50 g/L or >4 g/L.

- Radiology:

    - Early signs of ischaemia involving more than one-third of the middle cerebral artery territory demonstrated on brain CT scan.

Thrombolysis and Brain MRI

Brain CT scan is sufficient, especially when it is performed very soon after the onset of symptoms (recommendations based on CT scan). CT eliminates cerebral haemorrhage or another non-vascular cause for the symptoms.

No validated MRI criteria to define the indications for intravenous thrombolysis, but MRI should be preferred when it is available as first-line imaging procedure.

- Advantages of MRI compared to CT:

  - positive diagnosis of definite infarction;
  - precise visualization of the extent of ischaemia and possibly the ischaemic "penumbra";
  - visualization of the arterial occlusion.

- Disadvantages:

  - longer acquisition time;
  - contraindications;
  - absence of validated criteria for contraindications (apart from recent or old cerebral haemorrhage). It sometimes makes treatment decisions more difficult (micro bleeds, absence of visible arterial occlusion).

Special Cases

- Pregnant women, children less than 18 years old: no recommendation as excluded from clinical trials. Case by case assessment.
- Patients over the age of 80: IV thrombolysis can be considered within the first 3 h (HAS guideline—off-label).
- Seizure: does not constitute a real contraindication when ischaemia is documented (value of diffusion-weighted MRI).
- Cervical artery dissection without intracranial extension is not a contraindication.
- Procedure
- rt-PA (alteplase: Actilyse®) must be prescribed by a neurologist or a physician with a specialist diploma in Neurovascular Disease. Treatment must be administered in a unit allowing continuous monitoring of the patient's neurological status and blood pressure, preferably in a neurovascular unit.
- Discuss the risk/benefit balance of thrombolysis with the family and the patient prior to initiation of treatment.
- The patient's general condition must be assessed, including respiratory, cardiac and haemodynamic conditions. Meningitis or endocarditis must be excluded in the presence of fever.
- Neurological assessment is essential to assess severity (NIHSS).
- Emergency laboratory tests to exclude contraindications to thrombolysis, CT scan or MRI.
- Emergency CT scan or MRI (positive diagnosis; eliminate contraindications to thrombolysis).
- After obtaining consent from the patient or his/her next of kin, rt-PA may be administered: 0.9 mg/kg (10 % of dose by IV bolus injection, then the rest by slow IV injection over 1 h, not exceeding 90 mg). Blood pressure must be monitored regularly, every 15 min for 3 h, then every 30 min for 6 h and finally every 60 min for 24 h.
- Antiplatelet and heparin therapies are contraindicated within the first 24 h following the injection.

Complications

- Cerebral haemorrhage (symptomatic in 6–8 % of cases) (Figs. 14.3, 14.4, and 14.5).
- Risk factors: severe neurological deficit, early CT signs involving more than one-third of the middle cerebral artery territory, lesion on diffusion-weighted images >100 ml, mass effect, age >80 years, high blood pressure, diabetes and/or hypoglycaemia, platelet count <150,000/mm^3, protocol violation, other causes of haemorrhage: microbleeds, very low ADC, atrial fibrillation, heart failure, prior platelet antiaggregant therapy.
- Systemic haemorrhage.
- Allergy.
- Angioneurotic oedema.

Intra-Arterial Thrombolysis and Mechanical Thrombectomy (Figs. 14.6 and 14.7)

The clinical outcome after IV thrombolysis is less favourable in the case of proximal occlusion of a cerebral artery than in the case of more distal occlusion. The early recanalisation rate after IV thrombolysis is lower when the clot is situated in a large proximal artery.

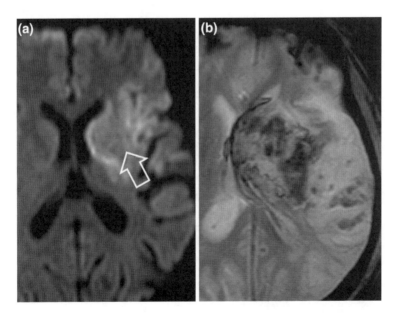

Fig. 14.3 Early complication of intravenous thrombolysis. Patient with infarction in the deep middle cerebral artery territory (**a** diffusion-weighted sequence, *hollow arrow*). Deterioration of neurological deficit following intravenous thrombolysis associated with reperfusion haematoma of the infarcted territory, hypointense on the T2*-weighted sequence (**b**)

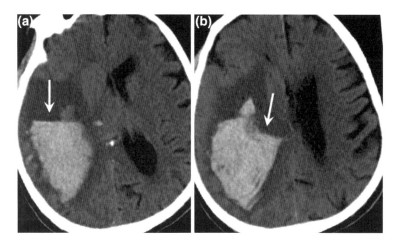

Fig. 14.4 Right parieto-occipital haematoma on CT scan in a patient after IV thrombolysis. Note the characteristic appearance of the haematoma with a fluid level (**a** and **b** *arrow*) related to hypodense noncoagulated blood lying on top of the hyperdense coagulated blood

Indications

Endovascular treatments may be indicated in certain circumstances, although no study has demonstrated the benefit of this treatment in the acute management of cerebral infarction. Endovascular treatment may be considered in the case of severe stroke with a NIHSS score ≥10.

IA Thrombolysis

- Beyond the time limit >4.5 h for IV thrombolysis and <6 h after the onset of symptoms for carotid artery thrombosis.
- Beyond the time limit >4.5 h for IV thrombolysis and <8 h after the onset of symptoms for vertebrobasilar thrombosis. rt-PA (Actilyse®) by slow infusion into the blood clot with a maximum dose of 20 mg. The infusion must last several minutes possibly by using an infusion pump (0.5–1 mg/min). IA thrombolysis and the IV + IA thrombolysis combination (±thrombectomy) increase recanalisation rates, but their clinical benefits are still under evaluation.

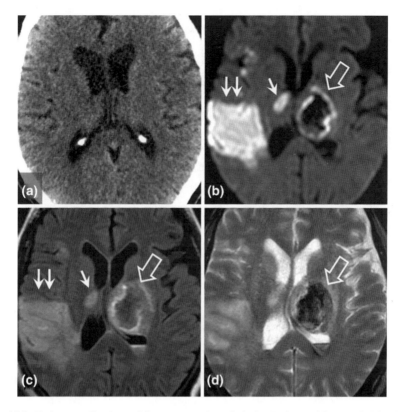

Fig. 14.5 Early complication of intravenous thrombolysis. Patient with superficial middle cerebral artery an infarction with normal early imaging less than 3 h after onset of symptoms (**a** CT). Deterioration of neurological deficit after intravenous thrombolysis associated with contralateral thalamic haematoma, hypointense on diffusion-weighted and T2*-weighted sequences (**b** and **d** *hollow arrows*) and isointense on FLAIR images (**c** *hollow arrow*). The superficial middle cerebral artery infarction is clearly visible on the follow-up MRI (**b** and **c** *double arrows*) with focal deep involvement (**b** and **c** *simple arrows*)

Mechanical Thrombectomy

- Second-line treatment, after failure of IV thrombolysis and <6 h after the onset of symptoms.
- For first-line treatment:
    - contraindication to IV or IA thrombolysis;
    - IV thrombolysis time limit > 4.5 h and < 6 h after the onset of symptoms, when blood clot is visible on imaging in a proximal trunk: terminal internal carotid artery, M1 segment or basilar artery (up to 8 h after onset of symptoms for the basilar artery).

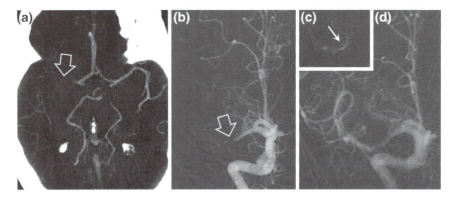

Fig. 14.6 65-year-old female patient with left hemiplegia for past 2 h due to cardioembolic stroke. CT angiography shows a nonopacified thrombosis of the right MCA (**a** *hollow arrow*). Arteriography confirms occlusion of the right middle cerebral artery bifurcation (**b** *hollow arrow*, right carotid arteriography, frontal view). Infusion of 7 mg of rt-PA (**c** *arrow*, microcatheter for infusion positioned in the clot) allowed thrombolysis and recanalisation (**d** follow-up right carotid artery arteriography after thrombolysis)

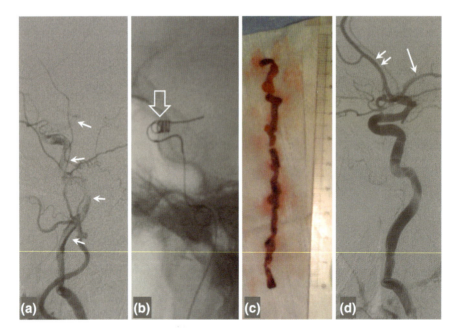

Fig. 14.7 72-year-old female patient with atherothrombotic occlusion of the left internal carotid artery (**a** *arrows*, absence of opacification of the left internal carotid artery on the arteriogram, lateral view) responsible for right hemiplegia and disorders of consciousness. The thrombectomy system was inserted into the internal carotid artery (**b** *hollow arrow*, system deployed) allowing removal of the clot after 3 passages of the system (**c** picture of the reconstituted clot). The final angiography shows recanalisation of the left internal carotid artery and opacification of the ACA (**d** *double arrows*) and left MCA (**d** *simple arrow*)

Appendix 1

NIHSS scale: measures the neurological deficit at the acute phase of ischaemic stroke. Completion time less than 7 min. Validated reproducible tool. Score during the first hours is correlated with long-term disability.

NIHSS Score

1a	**Level of consciousness**	Alert	0
		Not alert, but arousable by minor stimulation (question or command)	1
		Not alert (response to pain)	2
		Responds only with reflex motor or autonomic effects or totally unresponsive	3
1b	**LOC questions**	Answers both questions correctly	0
	Patient's age, the month	Answers one question correctly	1
	Only the initial answer is graded	Answers neither question correctly	2
1c	**LOC commands**	Performs both tasks correctly	0
	Open and close eyes, grip and release non-paretic hand.	Performs one task correctly	1
	Pantomime is Possible.	Performs neither task correctly	2
2	**Best Gaze**	Normal	0
	Horizontal eye movements or doll's eyes	Partial gaze palsy but able to cross midline	1
		Forced deviation or total gaze paresis	2
3	**Visual fields**	No visual loss	0
	Test by confrontation or visual threat as appropriate	Partial hemianopsia	1
		Complete hemianopsia	
		Bilateral hemianopsia, blindness	2
			3
4	**Facial paralysis**	Normal	0
	Noxious stimulus if necessary	Minor paralysis	1
		Partial paralysis	2
		Complete paralysis (upper and lower face)	3
5a	**Left motor arm**	No drift	0
	Left arm extended **for 10 s** at 90° in sitting position or at 45° in supine position	Drift (but does not hit bed before 10 s)	1
		Some effort against gravity (but drifts down to bed before 10 s)	2
		No effort against gravity, limb falls	3
		No movement	4
		Untestable (amputation, joint fusion, fracture, etc.)	X

(continued)

(continued)

5b	Right motor arm	No drift	0
	Right arm extended **for** **10 s** at 90° in sitting position or at 45° in supine position	Drift (but does not hit bed before 10 s)	1
		Some effort against gravity (but drifts down to bed before 10 s)	2
		No effort against gravity, limb falls	3
		No movement	4
		Untestable (amputation, joint fusion, fracture, etc.)	X
6a	Left motor leg	No drift	0
	Left leg extended **for 5 s** at 30° in supine position	Drift (but does not hit bed before 5 s)	1
		Some effort against gravity (but drifts down to bed before 5 s)	2
		No effort against gravity, leg falls to bed immediately	3
		No movement	4
		Untestable (amputation, joint fusion, fracture, etc.)	X
6b	**Right motor leg**	No drift	0
	Right leg extended **for 5 s** at 30° in supine position	Drift (but does not hit bed before 5 s)	1
		Some effort against gravity (but drifts down to bed before 5 s)	2
		No effort against gravity, leg falls to bed immediately	3
		No movement	4
		Untestable (amputation, joint fusion, fracture, etc.)	X
7	**Limb ataxia**	Absent	0
	Finger-nose-finger and heel-shin tests	Present in one limb	1
		Present in two limbs	2
	Assessed according to weakness	Untestable (paralysis, amputation, fracture, etc.)	X
8	**Sensory**	Normal	0
	Use pinprick to test face, arms, trunk, legs	Mild-to-moderate sensory loss	1
	Noxious stimulus if necessary	Severe to total sensory loss	2
9	**Best language**	No aphasia	0
	Name items, describe an image, read sentences	Mild-to-moderate aphasia (can be understood)	1
		Severe aphasia	2
		Mute, global aphasia	3

(continued)

(continued)

10	**Dysarthria**	Normal	0
	Ask patient to read an adequate sample of speech	Mild-to-moderate dysarthria (can be understood)	1
		Severe dysarthria (unintelligible), mute	2
		Untestable (intubated, other physical barrier)	X
11	**Extinction and Inattention**	No abnormality	0
	Simultaneous stimulus visual, tactile, auditory, spatial inattention or extinction	Visual, tactile, auditory, spatial or personal inattention	1
		Profound hemi-inattention or extinction to more than one modality	2
TOTAL			

Appendix 2

ASPECTS: Alberta Stroke Program Early CT Score is a 10-points quantitative topographic CT scan score.

For ASPECTS, the territory of the middle cerebral artery is allotted 10 points (fig. A-2.1). One point is subtracted for an area of early ischemic change for each of the defined regions. ASPECTS value is 10 points in a normal CT scan and 0 in diffuse ischemia throughout the territory of the middle cerebral artery.

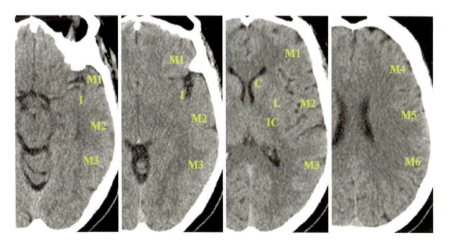

Fig. A.2.1 MCA territory regions as defined by ASPECTS. C- Caudate, I- Insular ribbon, IC-Internal Capsule, L- Lentiform nucleus, M1- Anterior MCA cortex, M2- MCA cortex lateral to the insular ribbon, M3- Posterior MCA cortex, M4, M5, M6 are the anterior, lateral and posterior MCA territories immediately superior to M1, M2 and M3, rostral to basal ganglia. Subcortical structures are allotted 3 points (C, L, and IC). MCA cortex is allotted 7 points (I, M1, M2, M3, M4, M5 and M6)

Within the first 3 hours of MCA stroke onset, ASPECTS values correlate inversely with the severity of NIHSS and functional outcome.

APSECTS value ≤7 are correlated with poor functional outcome and symptomatic intracerebral hemorrhage.

ASPECTS applied to un-enhanced CT-scans suggest that ASPECTS value ≥8 were associated with a greater benefit from i.v. thrombolysis.

Selected References

1. Barber PA et al. (2000) Validity and reliability of a quantitative computed tomography score in predicting outcome of hyperacute stroke before thrombolytic therapy. ASPECTS Study Group. Alberta Stroke Programme Early CT Score. Lancet. 355(9216):1670–1674
2. Demchuk AM et al (2005) NINDS rtPA Stroke Study Group, NIH. Importance of early ischemic computed tomography changes using ASPECTS in NINDS rtPA Stroke Study. Stroke. 36(10):2110-2115
3. Dzialowski I et al (2006) Extent of early ischemic changes on computed tomography (CT) before thrombolysis: prognostic value of the Alberta Stroke Program Early CT Score in ECASS II. Stroke. 37(4):973-978
4. The National Institute of Neurological Disorders and Stroke rt-PA Stroke Study Group (1995) Tissue plasminogen activator for acute ischemic stroke. N Engl J Med 333(24):1581–1587
5. Hacke W et al (1998) Randomised double-blind placebo-controlled trial of thrombolytic therapy with intravenous alteplase in acute ischaemic stroke (ECASS II). Second European-Australasian acute stroke study investigators. Lancet 352:1245–1251
6. Hacke W et al. ATLANTIS Trials Investigators; ECASS Trials Investigators; NINDS rt-PA Study Group Investigators (2004) Association of outcome with early stroke treatment: pooled analysis of ATLANTIS, ECASS, and NINDS rt-PA stroke trials. Lancet 363:768–774
7. Hacke W et al. ECASS Investigators (2008) Thrombolysis with alteplase 3 to 4.5 hours after acute ischemic stroke. N Engl J Med 359:1317–1329
8. Rha JH, Saver JL (2007) The impact of recanalization on ischemic stroke outcome: a meta-analysis. Stroke 38:967–973
9. Wahlgren N et al. SITS-MOST investigators.et al (2007) Thrombolysis with alteplase for acute ischaemic stroke in the safe implementation of thrombolysis in stroke-monitoring study (SITS-MOST): an observational study. Lancet 369:275–282
10. Wardlaw JM et al (2003) Thrombolysis for acute ischaemic stroke. Cochrane Database Syst Rev CD000213
11. Zangerle et al (2007) Recanalization after thrombolysis in stroke patients: predictors and prognostic implications. Neurology 68:39–44

Printed by Printforce, the Netherlands

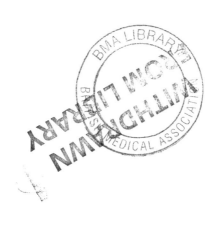
BMA LIBRARY

WITHDRAWN

BRITISH MEDICAL ASSOCIATION